Haematology

CLINICAL CASES UNCOVERED

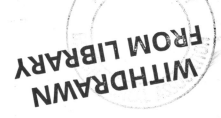
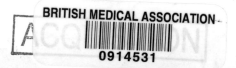

Haematology

CLINICAL CASES UNCOVERED

Shaun McCann

MB, FRCPI, FRCPath, FRCPEdin, Hon FTCD

Professor of Haematology
St James' Hospital, Dublin
and
University of Dublin
Trinity College, Ireland

Robin Foà

MD

Professor of Haematology
University 'La Sapienza'
Rome, Italy

Owen Smith

MA, MB, FRCPI, FRCPEdin, FRCPCH, FRCPath

Consultant Paediatric Haematologist
Our Lady's Hospital for Sick Children
Dublin, Ireland

Eibhlin Conneally

MB, PhD, MRCPI, FRCPath

Consultant Haematologist
St James' Hospital, Dublin
and
Lecturer in Haematology at the University of Dublin
Trinity College, Ireland

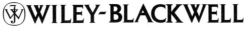

WILEY-BLACKWELL

A John Wiley & Sons, Ltd., Publication

Blackwell Publishing was acquired by John Wiley & Sons in February 2007. Blackwell's publishing program has been merged with Wiley's global Scientific, Technical and Medical business to form Wiley-Blackwell.

Registered office: John Wiley & Sons Ltd, The Atrium, Southern Gate, Chichester, West Sussex, PO19 8SQ, UK

Editorial offices: 9600 Garsington Road, Oxford, OX4 2DQ, UK
    The Atrium, Southern Gate, Chichester, West Sussex, PO19 8SQ, UK
    111 River Street, Hoboken, NJ 07030-5774, USA

For details of our global editorial offices, for customer services and for information about how to apply for permission to reuse the copyright material in this book please see our website at www.wiley.com/wiley-blackwell

Library of Congress Cataloging-in-Publication Data
Haematology / Shaun McCann . . . [et al.].
      p. ; cm. – (Clinical cases uncovered)
   Based on: Case-based haematology / Shaun McCann . . . [et al.]. 2005.
   Includes bibliographical references and index.
   ISBN 978-1-4051-8322-2
   1. Blood–Diseases–Case studies.   2. Hematology–Case studies.   I. McCann, Shaun R.
II. Case-based haematology.   III. Series.
   [DNLM: 1. Hematologic Diseases–diagnosis–Case Reports.   2. Diagnosis, Differential–Case Reports.   3. Hematologic Diseases–therapy–Case Reports.   WH 120 H134 2009]
   RC636.C37 2009
   616.1'5–dc22

                                                                                    2008039511

ISBN: 978-1-4051-8322-2

A catalogue record for this book is available from the British Library.

Set in 9 on 12 pt Minion by SNP Best-set Typesetter Ltd., Hong Kong
Printed and bound in Singapore by Fabulous Printers Pte Ltd

2   2009

Contents

(Part 3) Self-assessment, 162

Preface

This book is a development from *Case-Based Haematology*. We have added two didactic chapters, three new cases and a number of MCQs and SAQs to help you to assess your knowledge. This book is designed to make you think. I hope it will help you, not just in haematology, but in all areas of medicine.

The basis of medical practice is still listening and looking. This book is an attempt to make you do these things well and to ask for, and interpret, appropriate investigations. Remember Denis Burkitt, who with the simple tools of observation and listening, was able to make the seminal observation which resulted in the first description of cancer caused by an infectious agent. He had no elaborate tests or DNA analysis, just his eyes and ears.

You are not expected to know the answers to all the questions, especially in the first two chapters. However, I hope you will keep this book after you graduate as a doctor and refer to it in future years.

Medicine is a very privileged profession and a very interesting one. I hope this book helps you to be a better doctor and to enjoy your medical career, wherever it may take you.

Shaun McCann

Acknowledgements

I would like to acknowledge the contributions of my colleagues E.C, O.S, and R.F. I would also like to thank many other colleagues for their help, especially Dr Ronan McDermot, Professor Sean O'Briain, Professor Donald Weir, Dr Corrina McMahon, Mr David O'Brien, and Dr Emer Lawlor. Dr Ruth Gilmore and Dr Aileen Patterson are thanked for proof reading and helpful suggestions. My long time friend James Cogan provided illustrations but most importantly I am indebted to the patients who were enthusiastic about having their images used.

The original stimulus to developing a teaching manual came from my old boss and now friend Professor Harry Jacob from the University of Minnesota where I had my formative training in Haematology. To him and his associates I owe a huge debt.

How to use this book

Clinical Cases Uncovered (CCU) books are carefully designed to help supplement your clinical experience and assist with refreshing your memory when revising. Each book is divided into three sections: Part 1 Basics; Part 2 Cases; and Part 3 Self-assessment.

Part 1 gives a quick reminder of the basic science, history and examination, and key diagnoses in the area. Part 2 contains many of the clinical presentations you would expect to see on the wards or crop up in exams, with questions and answers leading you through each case. New information, such as test results, is revealed as events unfold and each case concludes with a handy case summary explaining the key points. Part 3 allows you to test your learning with several question styles

(MCQs, EMQs and SAQs), each with a strong clinical focus.

Whether reading individually or working as part of a group, we hope you will enjoy using your CCU book. If you have any recommendations on how we could improve the series, please do let us know by contacting us at: medstudentuk@oxon.blackwellpublishing.com.

Disclaimer

CCU patients are designed to reflect real life, with their own reports of symptoms and concerns. Please note that all names used are entirely fictitious and any similarity to patients, alive or dead, is coincidental.

Basic science

The cellular elements in the blood are continuously destroyed and replaced. What process is required to continuously replace them and keep the number of cells within well-defined limits?

The numbers of cells produced in an individual with a lifespan of 80–90 years is astronomical (12×10^6 granulocytes are produced each day). In order to maintain haemopoiesis throughout life, a pool of resting haemopoietic stem cells (HSCs) is required. These cells, given the appropriate stimulus, can differentiate along specific pathways and produce the mature cells of the peripheral blood. Because the pool of resting stem cells must be maintained at all times, these cells must be capable of self-replication and production of progeny. Each stem cell has the capacity to differentiate into any of the cells in the blood. Hence, these stem cells are 'pluripotent' and capable of self-renewal (Fig. 1).

Where else are HSCs found besides the bone marrow?

HSCs are found in very small numbers in the peripheral blood and in large numbers in umbilical cord blood. HSCs have the appearance of a small lymphocyte.

What tragic event served as a major stimulus to stem cell research?

Much of the research that led to our understanding of haemopoiesis came from the knowledge that ionizing radiation resulted in the death of experimental animals from infection or bleeding. Thus, the development of the atom bomb served as a stimulus for many experiments. This ultimately resulted in a therapeutic manoeuvre

Haematology: Clinical Cases Uncovered. By S. McCann, R. Foà, O. Smith and E. Conneally. Published 2009 by Blackwell Publishing, ISBN: 978-1-4051-8322-2

(allogeneic stem cell transplantation), which was to test all the theories of haemopoiesis.

How does stem cell transplantation verify the existence of pluripotent stem cells?

In animals, experiments can be carried out when the HSC donor is of a different sex from the recipient. The animal is initially exposed to irradiation in order to kill all the HSCs. The animal is then 'rescued' by injecting bone marrow cells from the donor. Haemopoiesis recovers but all of the haemopoietic cells in the bone marrow and blood of the recipient are derived from the donor. These survivors were called 'radiation chimaeras' after the mythological creature, which had the head of a lion, the body of a goat and the tail of a snake (Fig. 2). Human chimaeras are created when a patient receives HSCs from a healthy donor.

What are the names of the mature blood cells in the circulation?

Erythrocytes, neutrophils, eosinophils, basophils, monocytes (Fig. 3a–f) and platelets. Erythrocytes are derived from a nucleated cell in the bone marrow called a normoblast, which undergoes a number of divisions and extrudes its nucleus before being released into the blood. Granulocytes (neutrophils, eosinophils, basophils) and monocytes are likewise derived from a nucleated cell, but lymphocytes appear to be derived from a nucleated cell, which 'differentiates' at a very early stage. Platelets are derived from giant cells called megakaryocytes.

What test is commonly used clinically to measure the frequency of HSCs in humans?

There is no commonly used test available. It is estimated that HSCs occur at the frequency of 1 in 1 million nucleated cells in the bone marrow. Most laboratories depend on a test that measures the 'committed pool' of cells, i.e.

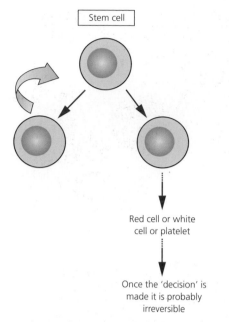

Stem cell

Red cell or white
cell or platelet

Once the 'decision' is
made it is probably
irreversible

Figure 1 A schematic illustration of self-renewing stem cells.

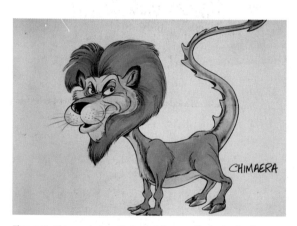

CHIMAERA

Figure 2 Chimaera. A mythological figure with the body of a goat, head of a lion and tail of a snake. First used when mice were successfully transplanted with haemopoietic stem cells. Now used in humans after stem cell transplant to denote cells of donor or recipient origin.

primitive cells that are already committed to a particular lineage such as a red cell or a granulocyte. Mononuclear cells from the bone marrow, umbilical cord blood or peripheral blood are put into a semi-solid supporting matrix and cytokines/growth factors are added. Following *in vitro* incubation for a variable number of days,

large groups of cells appear (colonies) and have the appearance of mature blood elements, e.g. red cells. Each colony represents growth from a single progenitor.

Figure 4 shows a colony of mature red cells and white cells known as a colony-forming unit – granulocyte, macrophage (CFU-GM). Figure 5 shows the different cell lineages and how they are measured. Each term, e.g. burst-forming unit – erythroid (BFU-E), refers to a colony of cells derived from a stem cell and which grows in the laboratory into a recognizable mature cell, in this case a red cell. Each colony is derived from a single stem cell.

The CD34 antigen (identified by flow cytometry) is an important clinical marker as it is a principal indicator of a pluripotent stem cell. It is expressed on haemopoietic stem cells and committed progenitor cells. The CD34$^+$ cell count is used to guide physicians when cells are being collected for stem cell transplantation.

How does a HSC differentiate into a mature blood cell?

The precise mechanism is unknown. However, it seems that cell–cell interactions (progenitors interact with mesenchymal cells in the bone marrow) and the expression of a large number of genes are important. Cytokines and growth factors may act in combination to activate signal transduction mechanisms. These intracellular factors activate the nucleus and stimulate the transcription of regulatory genes. These genes, in turn, influence proliferation, differentiation, apoptosis (programmed cell death) and development of mature cell function.

How can we recognize the potential for differentiation of HSCs?

HSCs and differentiating progenitors express antigens on their cell surface. The antigen type and frequency will change as the cell 'differentiates'. These antigens can be identified by a technique called 'flow cytometry'. The expression of different antigens allows us to identify progenitors of different lineages and to chart the development and differentiation of blood cells.

> **KEY POINT**
>
> The type of cell, i.e. its lineage, can be determined by the antigens on its surface. In many malignancies there is an accumulation of normal antigens in abnormal amounts.

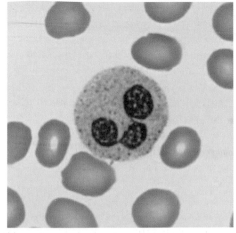

(a)

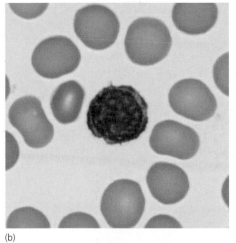

(b)

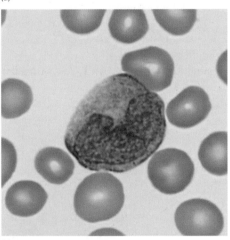

(c)

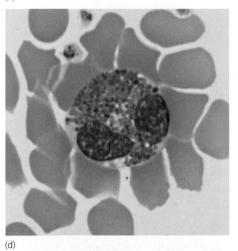

(d)

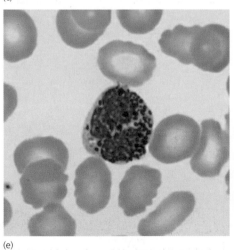

(e)

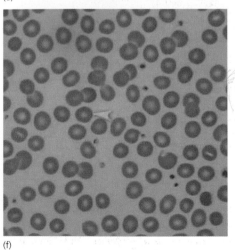

(f)

Figure 3 (a) Neutrophil, (b) lymphocyte, (c) monocyte, (d) eosinophil, (e) basophil and (f) normal erythrocyte.

Flow cytometry, or immunophenotyping, is made possible by the use of flow cytometers using the principle of hydrodynamic focusing (Fig. 6). The sample is injected, forcing the cell into the centre of the stream. As the cells intercept the light source they scatter the light and fluorochromes are excited to a higher energy state. This energy is released as a photon of light. The flow cytometer measures fluorescence per cell. After the different signals or pulses are amplified they are processed by an analogue to digital converter (ADC), which in turn allows for events to be plotted on a graphical scale (Fig. 7).

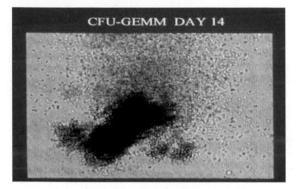

Figure 4 A colony of red cells and neutrophils grown in the laboratory and derived from a single stem cell.

Which cytokines or growth factors commonly found in the blood are available for clinical use?
Erythropoietin

Erythropoietin (EPO), a polypeptide, is the best known and is the main cytokine involved in erythrocyte differentiation, proliferation and apoptosis. It is largely produced in the kidney (Case 16). EPO production responds to hypoxia via a transcription factor complex called hypoxia inducible factor 1 (HIFI). A recombinant form is available and is used in the treatment of the anaemia of renal failure.

Granulocyte colony-stimulating factor

Granulocyte colony-stimulating factor (G-CSF) and granulocyte–macrophage colony-stimulating factor (GM-CSF) are glycopeptides and are secreted by granulocytes, monocytes, T lymphocytes, fibroblasts and endothelial cells. These growth factors are responsible for the production of granulocytes (G-CSF), granulocytes, eosinophils and monocytes (GM-CSF). The recombinant form of G-CSF is used in the treatment of congenital neutropenia and to 'mobilize' stem cells from the bone marrow into the peripheral circulation where they can be easily collected and used for stem cell transplantation.

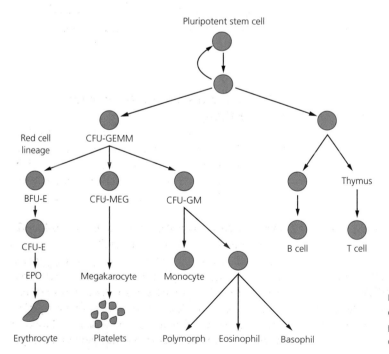

Figure 5 A schematic illustration of the different cell types, all derived from a pluripotent stem cell. Individual terms are defined in the Glossary.

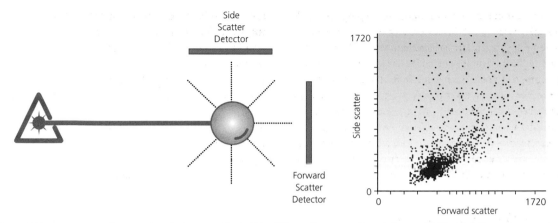

Figure 6 Flow cytometry or immunophenotyping, a method of identifying antigens on cells and thus establishing their lineage.

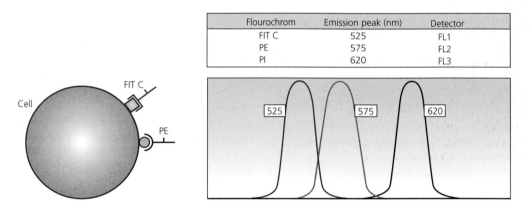

Flourochrom	Emission peak (nm)	Detector
FIT C	525	FL1
PE	575	FL2
PI	620	FL3

Figure 7 Flow cytometry or immunophenotyping showing the identification of antigens on cell surface using antibodies labelled with fluorochromes.

Thrombopoietin

Thrombopoietin (TPO) is a glycoprotein produced by the liver. It stimulates stem cell and platelet production. Newer formulations of recombinant TPO should soon be available to treat thrombocytopenia.

Stem cell factor

Stem cell factor is a glycoprotein produced by stromal cells and binds to the receptor c-Kit. It is essential for stem cell differentiation and proliferation.

How does apoptosis (programmed cell death) affect haemopoietic cells?

Apoptosis (programmed cell death) is a complex event, which terminates with the activation of caspases, DNA fragmentation and phagocytosis.

What is meant by the term stem cell plasticity?

Under experimental circumstances human pluripotent haemopoietic stem cells may be made to differentiate into non-haemopoietic tissues of mesenchymal origin such as muscle or cartilage. Whether this phenomenon can be reproduced in patients is unclear to date.

What major events occur during red cell (erythrocyte) development?

Fetal erythropoiesis develops in the yolk sac perhaps from a common progenitor with the endothelial cell known as the haemangioblast. The liver then predominates as the site of haemopoiesis followed by a period when the cells circulate and finally in the last 3 months of fetal life the bone marrow predominates as the major site of haemopoiesis. Haemoglobin (Hb) synthesis in fetal life differs from childhood and adult Hb (Case 8). It seems that undifferentiated stem cells contain most of the genes associated with the different cell lineages but over time many genes become silent and others are transcribed at a higher level. The first recognizable red cell precursor is a nucleated 'normoblast'. Following cell division these cells become smaller, develop haemoglobinized cytoplasm and eventually extrude their nucleus. A mature erythrocyte is a non-nucleated biconcave disc.

As red cells precursors mature, gene expression is up-regulated for blood group antigens, membrane proteins, glycolytic and haem synthetic enzymes. The final two steps are the synthesis of globin chains and haem. About 2% of circulating red cells are non-nucleated but not biconcave discs. They are larger than mature red cells, contain ribosomes and synthesize small amounts of Hb. They are called reticulocytes and mature into erythrocytes after about 48 hours.

KEY POINTS

Red cell lifespan is 120 days. Erythrocyte production rate is approximately 10^{10} per hour. EPO is the most important growth factor. EPO, following any hypoxic stimulus, binds to trans-membrane receptors and triggers a signalling system that results in red cell proliferation and inhibition of apoptosis. A critical factor is the activation of the JAK-2 kinase. Mutations in JAK-2 are now fundamental to our understanding of diseases in which proliferation of red cells, white cells and platelets predominate (Case 16).

What is the main function of the immune system and what cells predominate?

The immune system has a fundamental function in regulating defence mechanisms against foreign attacks, primarily infective agents. In addition, it also has an important role in the development of cancers (malignancy). The effectors of the immune system are represented by lymphocytes. We identify and recognize different types of lymphocytes (known as subsets) which have various intrinsic functional properties.

Lymphocytes with different functions originate from pluripotent stem cells. Humoral responses are mediated by B lymphocytes through their capacity to produce and secrete specific antibodies.

Cell-mediated immunity is regulated by T lymphocytes. During the process of physiologic development, common lymphocyte progenitors, which are derived from pluripotent stem cells, differentiate in lymphoid organs, including fetal liver and bone marrow in the case of B lymphocytes and the thymus for T lymphocytes. There is a third population of lymphocytes named natural killer (NK) cells which mediate responses against virus-infected and tumour cells.

What was the major discovery that allowed us to unravel the functional subsets of lymphocytes in the human immune system?

The turning point was the development of the monoclonal antibody (MoAb) technology in 1975 by Köhler and Milstein (who later won the Nobel Prize for Medicine) which rapidly led to the production of MoAbs directed against antigens expressed by different lymphocyte subsets (B, T, NK). This collection of antigens is known as the 'immunophenotypic' profile.

MoAbs were grouped according to the antigen identified. Thus, all the MoAbs directed against a well-defined antigen are identified according to a cluster of differentiation (CD). A table showing the MoAbs frequently used to identify different lymphocyte subsets is shown in the Appendix.

What laboratory technique is used to identify lymphocyte subsets?

Flow cytometry (Fig. 8).

What is the major function of B lymphocytes?

B lymphocytes are important in 'humoral immunity'. They produce antibodies also called immunoglobulins (Igs). These are glycoproteins that bind to specific antigens, neutrophils, lymphocytes and basophils. The antigen is initially processed by antigen presenting cells (APCs, monocytes and macrophages) and T cells are activated. In turn, the B lymphocyte proliferates and differentiates into a plasma cell, which produces specific antibody which will destroy or opsonize the antigen.

What is meant by the term opsonization?

Opsonization is when antibodies make a pathogen ready for digestion.

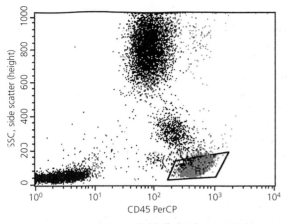

Figure 8 A dot plot of white cells labelled with an antibody to CD45 (green), an antigen present on all white cells.

Table 1 B-cell surface antigens at different stages of differentiation.

Immature B cells	CD10 (CALLA)
B cells beginning heavy chain rearrangement	CD19, TdT
B cells beginning light chain rearrangement	CD20, surface Ig

CALLA, common acute lymphoblastic leukaemia antigen; Ig, immunoglobulin; TdT, terminal deoxynucleotidyl transferase.

How do B cells recognize antigens and produce specific antibodies?

Each antibody (Ig) molecule has two heavy and two light chains. During early development in the bone marrow the genes for heavy and light chains are rearranged in that order. Once rearrangement is complete, the cell will express the antibody molecule on its surface. Mature B lymphocytes express IgM and IgD on their cell surface, which is important for cell survival. The cell surface antigen profile is shown in Table 1. Maturing B lymphocytes leave the bone marrow and migrate to lymph nodes where they congregate in an area called the germinal centre. Having recognized an antigen by binding to it, the B lymphocyte then undergoes a process called somatic hypermutation, i.e. mutations (rearrangements) occur in the variable region genes. The cells will divide and proliferate into plasma cells or B memory cells and produce specific antibody, as shown in Table 1.

How do T cells exert their function?

T cells are important in 'cell mediated immunity'. T-cell maturation occurs in the thymus. There are four T-cell receptor (TCRs) genes: α, β, γ and δ. Like in the B lymphocyte, the TCR genes undergo rearrangement so that a mature T cell will only express α/β or γ/δ (5%) receptors on its surface. The TCR recognizes a major histocompatibility complex (MHC) molecule and the T cell leaves the thymus. T memory cells provide the immune system with a memory so that these cells will rapidly proliferate if subsequently exposed to the same antigen.

What major events take place during white blood cell development?

Granulocytes are white blood cells (WBCs), neutrophils, eosinophils and basophils found in the circulation. Granulocytes are derived from haemopoietic stem cells in the bone marrow under the influence of cytokines (G-CSF is the most important). Neutrophils have a lifespan of around 7 hours in the circulation and leave the circulation as part of the inflammatory reaction. There is a large reserve of granulocyte precursors in the bone marrow. Normal individuals can increase the production of WBCs by 10–20 times. Approximately 50% of the granulocytes and monocytes are 'marginating', i.e. adherent to the sidewall of blood vessels but are 'available' if required. The predominant granulocyte is the neutrophil and its function is phagocytosis of microorganisms.

> **KEY POINT**
>
> Following bacterial infection, neutrophils are attracted by chemotactic factors. Neutrophils ingest antibody and complement-coated bacteria to form a phagosome. The neutrophil degranulates and various enzymes are released. H_2O_2 is produced and interacts with O_2^- in the presence of iron to generate singlet oxygen and hydroxyl radicals, both of which are toxic to bacteria.

What other types of granulocytes are present in the circulation?

Eosinophils and basophils are also derived from haemopoietic stem cells in the bone marrow. Eosinophils are important in the response to parasitic infection, allergy and drug reactions. Basophils are also implicated in allergy and drug reactions.

What other WBCs besides granulocytes are important and what is their function?

Monocytes are also derived from a haemopoietic stem cell in the bone marrow under the influence of the cytokine GM-CSF and are very closely related to granulocytes. They have a similar phagocytic and killing function (enhanced by GM-CSF), and are found in the spleen and liver as well as the circulation.

What other cells are found in the blood besides erythrocytes and white cells?

Platelets. These are very small non-nucleated structures derived from the 'shedding' of the cytoplasm of giant cells in the bone marrow called megakaryocytes. Megakaryocytes are polyploid (increased DNA content) and have multilobed nuclei. Unlike other bone marrow cells, megakaryocytes become larger as they mature. Platelets have a lifespan of about 7 days.

What is the function of platelets?

The principal function of platelets is to enhance the generation of thrombin (blood clotting). They do this by acting as a catalytic surface. The important structural elements of this catalytic surface include: (i) plasma membranes rich in glycoproteins and phospholipids; and (ii) secretory granules. The plasma membrane is a highly reactive surface on which haemostatic (procoagulation and anticoagulation) reactions can take place.

The plasma membrane is predominantly in deep invaginations and the main glycoproteins are GP IIb–IIIa (the most plentiful). GP IIb–IIIa acts as a receptor for fibrinogen. GP Ib–IX–V is the major von Willebrand receptor and binding is the initial step that localizes platelets to the site of vascular injury.

The phospholipids in the platelet membrane provide the surface to mediate Ca^{2+} dependent binding of vitamin K dependent coagulation factors through their γ-carboxyglutamic acid residues.

Platelet granules (α granules, dense granules and lysosomes) contribute to platelet adhesion and aggregation, and to blood clotting. For a diagram and explanation of blood clotting see Case 18.

KEY POINT

Platelet adhesion and aggregation are sufficient to stop bleeding from small vessels. Coagulation factor activation and fibrin formation, together with platelet aggregation and adhesion, are required to stop bleeding from larger wounds.

Approach to the patient

Many patients are seen initially in a primary care setting and may have vague symptoms. In the hospital the majority of patients are referred for investigation and expert opinion because of abnormal blood test results. Others are referred to the haematologist because abnormal blood test results occur during the diagnosis or management of another apparently unrelated condition.

As always, the most important diagnostic event is the history-taking.

What should be your initial interaction with the patient?

In an ambulatory patient it is important to observe the patient's general demeanour and ease of movement. It is important to greet the patient by asking their name while offering to shake hands at the same time. (In some cultures it is impolite for a man to shake hands with a woman.) You should introduce yourself by your full name and title.

Why is it important to observe the patient and what can you learn from a handshake?

You can observe if the gait is steady and if the patient is in pain when they walk. An unsteady gait might suggest a peripheral neuropathy or subacute degeneration of the spinal cord seen in vitamin B_{12} deficiency (Case 3). Pain may be bony and reflect malignant disease or a fracture such as in multiple myeloma. A dorsal kyphosis should also arouse the same suspicion (Case 13). A handshake provides information about the patient's state of mind. Excessive sweating may be the result of nervousness or hyperthyroidism. Rheumatoid disease and other forms of arthritis may be evident. As you shake hands you can

carry out a rapid general inspection noting the presence of jaundice, seen in haemolysis or cyanosis, or plethora in erythrocytosis.

Why should you ask the patient their name?

Although you might know the patient's name it is important to ask. First, simply to make sure the patient you are interviewing is who you think he/she is. Secondly, to test the patient's memory and ability to understand and speak. Providing the patient with their name and asking for confirmation is not adequate as he/she might affirm without understanding the question. Chronic alcoholism, multiple small strokes, Alzheimer's disease or vitamin B_{12} deficiency can impair memory or understanding.

Why should you introduce yourself by name and title?

It is important for the patient to know your name as it provides a sense of security and gives the patient confidence. Your title is important as it also lets the patient know precisely with whom they are dealing. Never call a patient by their first name unless they ask you to as it conveys disrespect or over-familiarity. You can be friendly and put the patient at their ease without using first names.

Frequently a patient will ask you if they may bring a spouse, relative or friend into the interview. What should be your response?

Gently but firmly you should deny the request. A second person can often inhibit the patient from revealing certain details about their complaint to avoid embarrassment. Likewise you could be inhibited from asking certain questions. Tell the patient that it would be perfectly acceptable to bring in their friend/relative at the end of the interview when you can explain the probable

Haematology: Clinical Cases Uncovered. By S. McCann, R. Foà, O. Smith and E. Conneally. Published 2009 by Blackwell Publishing, ISBN: 978-1-4051-8322-2

diagnosis and what further steps should be taken. This also provides you with an opportunity to corroborate parts of the history, which might have appeared unclear.

What should be done next?

You should ask the patient to tell you, in their own words, why they have come to see you. Be patient. Do not rush the patient or give the impression you are in a hurry. However, do not let the patient wander off and gently but firmly steer them back to their story.

> **KEY POINT**
>
> Remember history-taking is the most important interaction between the doctor and the patient. At the completion of the history a differential diagnosis should be made. A small number of diagnoses will be made when an unexpected physical sign is uncovered during the examination. Even more rarely will performing laboratory tests make an unsuspected diagnosis.

What should be done after the patient has completed his/her story?

Find out how long the complaint has been present, the approximate starting date of the symptoms (it may be useful to link the starting date to a public holiday or a personal event such as the patient's birthday) and if the symptoms are getting worse or better. Does anything bring on or relieve them? (The pain of multiple myeloma is typically worse at night, whereas musculo-skeletal pain tends to be relieved by rest.) Are there any associated features, such as weight loss, fever or night sweats, which are often associated with haematological malignancies? A social history should be taken with particular attention to travel (infectious diseases, e.g. malaria, may have important haematological manifestations), recreational and illicit drugs, and proprietary medications or herbal remedies.

A family history should be taken of haematological malignancy, coeliac disease, abnormalities of haemoglobin synthesis (e.g. thalassaemia or sickle cell disease or other haemoglobinopathies), diseases of iron metabolism (e.g. haemochromatosis) and autoimmune diseases. The family history should include parents, siblings and children. Causes of death of grandparents should be

determined, if possible. A system review should be carried out and sexual practices should be ascertained.

> **KEY POINT**
>
> A symptom is what a patient complains of, e.g. a sore throat. A sign is what the doctor finds when he/she examines a patient, e.g. an infected pharynx.

What points on general examination of the haematological patient should you be especially alert to?

Note if the patient is jaundiced (icteric) by looking at the sclera as this might imply haemolysis of ineffective erythropoiesis. A bronze colour in the skin should not be confused with icterus or jaundice as it is usually caused by iron deposition and is seen in diseases such as haemochromatosis (Case 2). Cyanosis might suggest congenital heart disease or heart failure. A plethoric face suggests erythrocytosis and pallor (palmar creases or conjunctival membranes) is common in anaemia (Fig. 9). Spooning of the nails, koilonychia and cracking at the angles of the mouth are seen in severe iron deficiency (Case 1). An unusual cause of blood loss is hereditary telangiectasiae. These may be seen in the nail beds, lips and tongue while also occurring in the gastroenterological tract.

Purpura, bleeding into the skin, may reflect a low platelet count although in elderly people is often

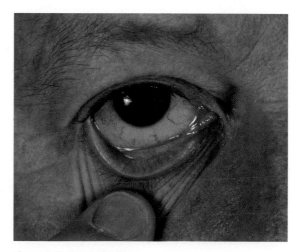

Figure 9 Conjunctival pallor.

present on the backs of the hands and is secondary to minor trauma together with loss of subcutaneous tissue (called senile purpura). Subconjunctival haemorrhages (Case 9, Fig 59) may result from a low platelet count and may be particularly prominent if the patient has vomited or has had a bout of coughing. Purpura does not blanch on pressure, unlike small dilated blood vessels. In chronic liver disease spider naevi may be present on the face, arms and trunk. These small dilated arterioles blanch under pressure and fill from the centre and are found in the drainage area of the superior vena cava.

> ### KEY POINT
>
> Before examining a patient, always explain what you are about to do in simple language, e.g. 'I would like to feel your tummy' rather than 'I would like to conduct a clinical examination of your abdomen'. Ask if the patient has any tenderness in the area to be examined and always observe the patient's face during the examination looking for signs of pain or discomfort. Reassure the patient that you will try not to hurt them.

What other physical signs might be present on general inspection?

Enlarged lymph nodes or tonsillar enlargements may be seen in the mouth and neck in haematological malignan-

cies. They may also be visible in the axillae and groins. Gum hypertrophy may be seen in leukaemia (Fig. 10).

How do you approach the examination of the lymph nodes?

First ask the patient if they have noticed any lumps or bumps when dressing or washing. Ask them to undress to the waist. The patient should sit on a couch or chair. Look into an open mouth for enlargement of the tonsils. Standing in front of the patient, look to see if there are any obvious masses in the neck. Examine the lymph nodes in the head and neck (Fig. 11). Ask the patient to

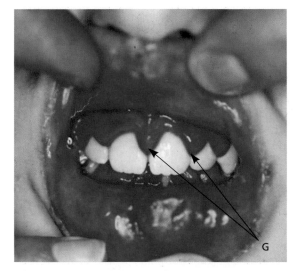

Figure 10 Gum hypertrophy (G).

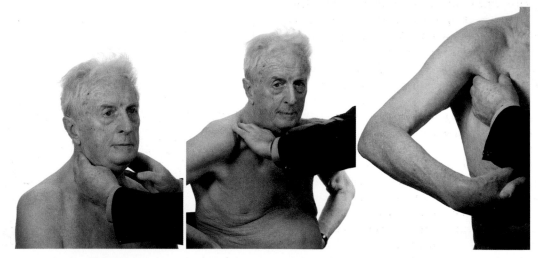

Figure 11 Examination of lymph nodes.

put their hands on their hips and move their elbows slightly forward. Assess the supraclavicular regions and then the axillae. Measure any enlarged lymph nodes and record size and the following characteristics: mobility, fixed or mobile; texture, hard or rubbery. Ask the patient to lie down and examine the inguinal nodes and record the characteristics above.

> **KEY POINT**
>
> Lymph node enlargement, which is painful, is usually inflammatory in nature. Lymph nodes that are immobile and painless are commonly malignant.

Which abdominal organs are most likely to be enlarged in haematological diseases?

The liver and spleen. Before estimating the size of these organs look at the abdomen, loins and the back for scars. The patient may have had a splenectomy, a kidney removed or other abdominal surgery, which could influence the haematological findings (e.g. a previous splenectomy could explain the signs of hyposplenism on the blood film).

To estimate the upper borders of the liver percuss the chest lightly from an area of resonance, over the lung, towards an area of dullness. When the percussion note changes mark the skin, with the patient's permission. This is usually in the 5th intercostal space. The lower border of the liver should be palpated, beginning from the right iliac fossa. The liver edge can be felt during inspiration and nodules may sometimes be detectable. Mark the lower border and measure the liver span in the mid-clavicular line. In an adult the span should be 12–15 cm. Do not comment on the size of the liver in 'fingers'.

The spleen may sometimes be visible protruding from below the left costal margin. Stand on the right-hand side, asks the patient to take a breath and observe. The spleen is not palpable or visible in a normal individual. Begin palpation from the right iliac fossa and proceed to the left hypochondrium as the patient is breathing. The enlarged spleen will move down freely with each inspiration. If the spleen is markedly enlarged the notch may be palpable on the medial border. The length of the spleen should be measured from the left costal margin, in quiet inspiration and recorded in centimeters.

What radiological investigations are commonly used in the evaluation of 'haematology patients'?

A radiograph of the chest, an ultrasound of the abdomen and a computed tomography (CT) scan of the chest and abdomen (Fig. 12). Remember, an ultrasound does *not* utilize radiation and a CT examination exposes the patient to the equivalent radiation dose to approximately 800 chest radiographs.

> **KEY POINT**
>
> The haematological examination is incomplete until the results of a full blood count are assessed and a blood film is examined microscopically.

What should be done next?

Explain to the patient, in ordinary language, what you think is wrong and how serious you think it is. Clarify what type of tests you recommend and precisely how they will be carried out and when the results are likely to be available. Ascertain if the patient understands what you have said. The best way to do this is to get the patient to explain to you, in their own words, what they have understood. Ask the patient if they would now like to bring in their friend/relative and go through the same procedure with them.

> **KEY POINT**
>
> In the case of an unconscious patient or one unable to give a history, a relative or friend who is familiar with the preceding events should be asked to provide the information.

What type of blood sample is required for routine analysis?

Blood taken into a tube containing the anticoagulant EDTA, a calcium chelator, is used in the majority of automated cell counters.

What parameters are commonly measured?

The number of red cells, their size/volume and haemoglobin content are measured. The percentage of

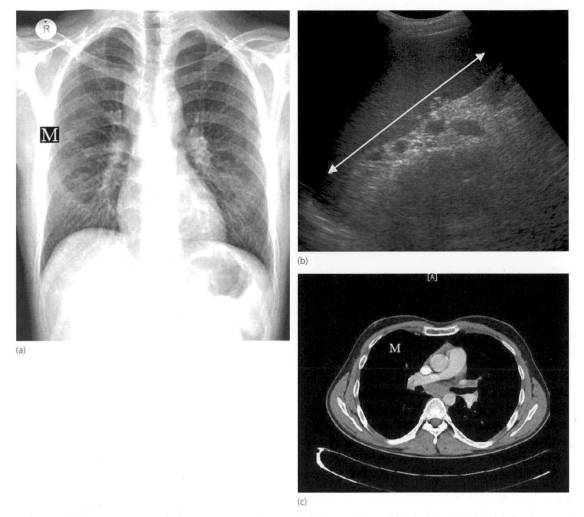

Figure 12 (a) Chest radiograph showing mediastinal lymphadenopathy (M). (b) An ultrasound showing an enlarged spleen. (c) A computed tomography (CT) scan showing mediastinal lymphadenopathy (M).

plasma is calculated. The total number of white blood cells and the number of granulocytes, monocytes, eosinophils, basophils, lymphocytes and platelets are counted.

Normal laboratory values may vary from laboratory to laboratory and country to country depending on the type of equipment used to carry out the assay and the population being tested. It is extremely important to check the reference values in the laboratory that is carrying out the test for your patient. The values given in Table 2 have been obtained from the laboratory from St. James's Hospital in Dublin and are in common use in Europe. Results given in brackets are those commonly used in North America.

What is the value of examining the blood film?

Microscopic examination of the blood film permits the evaluation of the shape, size and colour (usually reflects the degree of haemoglobinization) of the red blood cells. It facilitates detailed examination of the appearance of the white blood cells and platelets, and it allows the identification of abnormal cells, e.g. leukaemia cells (Fig. 13). It confirms the number and size of the platelets.

Table 2 Normal blood count values for adults.

	Normal range	
	Female	Male
Haemoglobin	11.5–16.4 g/dL	13.5–18.0 g/dL
Red cell count	$4.0–5.2 \times 10^{12}$/L (10^6/µL)	$4.6–5.7 \times 10^{12}$/L (10^6/µL)
MCV	83–99 fl (µm³)	
MCH	26.7–32.5 pg/cell	
MCHC	30.8–34.6 g/dL	
Platelet count	$140–450 \times 10^9$/L (10^3/µL)	
WBC	$4.0–11.0 \times 10^9$/L (10^3/µL)	
Neutrophils	$2.0–7.5 \times 10^9$/L (10^3/µL)	
Lymphocytes	$1.5–3.5 \times 10^9$/L (10^3/µL)	
Monocytes	$0.2–0.8 \times 10^9$/L (10^3/µL)	
Eosinophils	$0.04–0.40 \times 10^9$/L (10^3/µL)	
Reticulocytes	$14.0–100 \times 10^9$/L	
ESR*	1.0–30.0 mm/hour	1.0–22.0 mm/hour

ESR, erythrocyte sedimentation rate; MCH, mean corpuscular haemoglobin; MCHC, mean corpuscular haemoglobin concentration; MCV, mean corpuscular volume; WBC, white blood cell. *ESR measurement is automated. Male ranges as for females unless otherwise indicated.

> **KEY POINT**
>
> Blood taken in an EDTA container for evaluation should be considered in a similar fashion to a biopsy. In this case, it is a biopsy of a mesenchymal organ called blood but may yield information similar to that obtained from the biopsy of a solid organ.

APPROACH TO THE PAEDIATRIC HAEMATOLOGY PATIENT

In contrast to adults, a parent or carer almost invariably accompanies children.

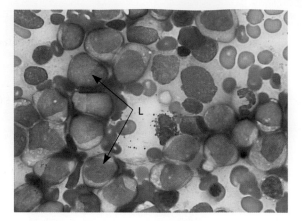

Figure 13 Blood film showing 'leukaemia blasts' (L) with large nuclei, prominent nucleoli and few other distinguishing features.

During the initial period of history-taking and clinical examination it is important to make the child and parent or carer feel relaxed. Observe the child for sweating, cough, dyspnoea and see if he/she is holding a position to protect a limb or other part of body. Is the child alert? Is the child sick? If the parent or carer says the child is sick they are usually correct. It should be stressed that children are not small adults and the history, physical examination and interpretation of the blood results will vary according to the age, race, family history and consanguinity of the child and parents (Table 3).

> **KEY POINT**
>
> Iron deficiency in adults should lead to an immediate search for blood loss, whereas in children nutritional aspects are far more important. What we see in children is far more likely to be caused by infection, poor nutrition or bleeding than to malignancy or rare disorders such as haemolytic anaemia.

How important is dietary history in assessing the cause of anaemia in children?

Dietary history is very important as it is related to a source of iron. Infants, particularly those delivered prematurely, and those consuming large amounts of cow's milk or formula unsupplemented with iron are at risk of iron deficiency anaemia as are children and adoles-

Table 3 Normal blood count values from birth to 18 years.

	Birth (term infants)	2 weeks	2 months	6 months	1 year	2–6 years	6–12 years	12–18 years (female)	12–18 years (male)
Haemoglobin (g/dL)	14.9–23.7	13.4–19.8	9.4–13.0	10.0–13.0	10.1–13.0	11.0–13.8	11.1–14.7	12.1–15.1	12.1–16.6
RBC × 10^{12}/L (10^6/µL)	3.7–6.5	3.9–5.9	3.1–4.3	3.8–4.9	3.9–5.1	3.9–5.0	3.9–5.2	4.1–5.1	4.2–5.6
Haematocrit (hct)	0.47–0.75	0.41–0.65	0.28–0.42	0.30–0.38	0.30–0.38	0.32–0.40	0.32–0.43	0.35–0.44	0.35–0.49
MCV fl (µm³)	100–125	88–110	84–98	73–84	70–82	72–87	76–90	77–94	77–92
WBC × 10^9/L (10^3/µL)	10.0–26.0	6.0–21	5.0–15	6.0–17	6.0–16	6.0–17	4.5–14.5	4.5–13	
Neutrophils × 10^9/L (10^3/µL)	2.7–14.4	1.5–5.4	0.7–4.8	1.0–6.0	1.0–8.0	1.5–8.5	1.5–8.0	1.5–6	
Lymphocytes × 10^9/L (10^3/µL)	2.0–7.3	2.8–9.1	3.3–10.3	3.3–11.5	3.4–10.5	1.8–8.4	1.5–5.0	1.5–4.5	
Monocytes × 10^9/L (10^3/µL)	0–1.9	0.1–1.7	0.4–1.2	0.2–1.3	0.2–0.9	0.15–1.3	0.15–1.3	0.15–1.3	
Eosinophils × 10^9/L (10^3/µL)	0.0–0.85	0.0–0.85	0.05–0.9	0.1–1.1	0.05–0.9	0.05–1.1	0.05–1.0	0.05–0.8	
Platelets × 10^9/L (10^3/µL)	150–450	170–500	210–650	210–560	200–550	210–490	170–450	180–430	

MCV, mean corpuscular volume; RBC, red blood cell count; WBC, white blood cell count. Male ranges as for females unless otherwise indicated.

cents who consume little meat. A history of pica (Case 1) suggests a possible iron deficiency, lead toxicity or both.

Breastfed infants or mothers who follow a strict vegan diet may become deficient in vitamin B_{12}.

Is it important to ask if the child was jaundiced at birth?

A neonatal history of jaundice (hyperbilirubinanaemia) supports a possible diagnosis of congenital haemolytic anaemia such as hereditary spherocytosis, which is further supported by a family history of anaemia, splenectomy and/or cholecystectomy (Case 5).

Is it important to ask if the child is taking any medication?

Medication history is pertinent in all patients as certain drugs can induce oxidative haemolysis (an enzymopathy, e.g. G6PD deficiency). Other medications may cause immune haemolysis, such as penicillin, or a decrease in red cell production, as with chloramphenicol, but the latter usually causes pancytopenia. A history of recent travel may suggest exposure to infections such as malaria.

Has the child ever passed red urine?

Haemoglobinuria may provide a clue to the cause of the anaemia. Possible factors include infection, medication and foods (fava beans in G6PD deficiency). Past medical history should enquire about neonatal jaundice, recurrent infections, arthritis, rash, mouth ulcers or thyroid disease suggesting autoimmune haemolysis. Family history should include ancestry (African, Mediterranean or Arab ancestry suggests G6PD deficiency, mainly but not exclusively in males, or sickle cell disease).

Of what importance is the age at which the child first had symptoms or signs?

Patients with α-thalassaemia major are symptomatic in the fetal or neonatal period and are common in South-East Asia, Mediterranean, Middle East, North and West Africa. A family history for iron deficiency that fails to respond to iron may be incorrect and an important pointer to the diagnosis of thalassaemia.

> **KEY POINT**
>
> Ask for the patient's ethnic origin as the thalassaemias, which are usually recessive, are common in South-East Asia, the Mediterranean, Middle East, North and West Africa. A family history of iron deficiency that fails to respond to iron replacement may be incorrect and an important pointer to the diagnosis of thalassaemia.

What is the differential diagnosis in a plethoric child?

A plethoric child will usually have elevated haemoglobin (erythrocytosis). The patient's age is very important as most children with polycythemia have congenital heart disease or severe lung disease. Symptoms or signs of pulmonary or cardiac disease, such as dyspnoea and cyanosis, may be critical pointers to the high haemoglobin levels. In neonates it is important to ask about delayed clamping of the umbilical cord, maternal diabetes or other causes of chronic fetal hypoxia. Dehydration is the most common cause of erythrocytosis (polycythaemia) as volume depletion increases the haematocrit. The polycythemia is corrected by rehydration.

What should you suspect in a child with recurrent infections?

The presence of unexpected infection affecting the skin, mucus membranes, perineum, lungs and abscess formation and/or failure to thrive suggests that the child may be neutropenic.

> **KEY POINT**
>
> Neutropenia is defined as a neutrophil count of $<1.5 \times 10^9$/L. However, a significant risk of serious infection is usually seen when the neutrophil count is $<0.5 \times 10^9$/L. In children of African descent the normal neutrophil count is lower than that in Caucasians.

What would you expect to find on clinical examination?

Failure to thrive or recent weight loss can be a presenting feature. Particular attention should be paid to examination of the ears, nose and throat (scarred tympanic membranes, gingivitis and aphthous ulceration, postnatal dip) respiratory tract (recurring cough, wheeze, chest deformity, cervical adenopathy), haemopoietic system (lymphadenopathy, hepatosplenomegaly and pallor) and skin (abscess, especially nail infections). Documentation of fevers is important, but rectal temperatures should be avoided because of the risk of causing Gram-negative bacteraemia.

How may a child present with a possible bleeding disorder?

Bleeding into the skin (petechial purpura/haematomas) from mucosal membranes (epistaxis, menorrhagia) or into joints (haemarthroses) or from the renal tract (haematuria) are the most common sites of blood loss in a child with a bleeding disorder.

> **KEY POINT**
>
> An incidental abnormal coagulation screen during presurgical screening should always be investigated prior to surgery.

How does the family history help in a child with a suspected bleeding disorder?

A family bleeding history in males suggests haemophilia A or B and the usual pattern consists of deep-seated haematomas or haemarthroses. The most common cause of inherited bleeding disorder in males and females is von Willebrand's disease where mucosal bleeding, especially nose bleeds and heavy periods (menorrhagia), are the most common manifestations.

What common acquired disorders cause bleeding into the skin (purpura)?

A palpable purpuric rash, usually in the lower limbs, suggests the vasculitis of Henoch–Schönlein purpura. Less well-localized rashes are commonly seen in viral infections, but an acutely ill child with a purpuric rash should be assumed to have meningococcal septicaemia. A purpuric rash, which becomes necrotic, indicates a diagnosis of purpura fulminans caused by viral or bacterial infection secondary to a deficiency of the natural anticoagulant protein C or S.

A non-palpable pruritic generalized rash suggests thrombocytopenia. This may be accompanied by bleeding into mucosal surfaces. A low platelet count does *not* cause haemarthrosis. In the absence of any other physical finding, such as lymphadenopathy or splenomegaly, a diagnosis of autoimmune thrombocytopenia is most likely. A blood film should always be carefully examined and if the diagnosis is in doubt a bone marrow aspirate should be examined. Children with acute leukaemia may present with purpura, but there are usually other abnormalities found when a blood film is examined.

In neonates, it should also be emphasized that obtaining a detailed maternal history, including bleeding problems, pre-eclampsia and drug ingestion in the present and past pregnancies and any history of viral infections (cytomegalovirus, rubella, herpes simplex and HIV) or connective tissue disease (systemic lupus erythematosus), will save time and investigations.

What are the common causes of enlarged lymph nodes in children?

Most of the illnesses manifesting with large lymph nodes represent common bacterial and viral infections, and tend to improve spontaneously or after appropriate antibiotic use. At the same time, enlarged lymph nodes can be an initial sign of a childhood malignancy.

How can the history help?

The character and time-course of the adenopathy are important. A rapid onset of unilateral groin adenopathy following trauma to the lower extremity suggests infection. In contrast, generalized adenopathy that has appeared over time in association with weight loss, fevers and night sweats suggest a haematological malignancy (lymphoma/leukaemia) or an infection such as tuberculosis.

> **KEY POINT**
>
> As in adults, tender lymphadenopathy in children is usually associated with an infective or inflammatory reaction while non-tender rubbery lymph node enlargement is more often seen with a malignant process.

Is the age of the child important when considering the differential diagnosis?

The age of the child with lymphadenopathy has a bearing on the differential diagnosis. It is extremely rare to see malignancy in neonates compared to older children and young adolescents. Lymphadenopathy in the neonatal period is most likely secondary to viral infections.

How important is the family and travel history in helping to make a diagnosis?

Family history should include place of birth and recent travel, the latter to determine whether the child has been exposed to geographical areas with high rates of infection such as kala azar, tuberculosis or histoplasmosis. There may be a family history of HIV infection or tuberculosis.

What other questions may be relevant?

Always ask about pets. If there are animals in the household they may play a significant part in the lymphadenopathy. The presence of cats or kittens (cat scratch fever, toxoplasmosis) which scratch the child are often omitted from the parent's history of the patient unless such questions are specifically asked.

Case 1 | A 35-year-old tired woman

Jenny Murphy is a 35-year-old Caucasian woman who works as a secretary. Over the last year she has noticed a decrease in her energy, which has become more marked in the last few months. Normally a very active person, she no longer goes hill walking or plays squash because she is 'too tired' at the end of the day.

Jenny has been living with her partner for 5 years and has never been pregnant. She smokes 10 cigarettes a day and drinks 5 units of alcohol weekly, usually at weekends. Her doctor carried out a blood test.

What could cause her symptoms?

She could have respiratory disease as she is a smoker but there is no history of cough or sputum. Cardiovascular disease could explain some of her symptoms but she is young with no history of cardiovascular symptoms preceding this episode. She could also be anaemic or depressed as the history is fairly non-specific.

| *The blood test shows that her haemoglobin is low.*

What type of anaemia is a 35-year-old Caucasian woman likely to have?

The most likely underlying mechanism in Jenny is iron deficiency, which is a common cause of anaemia, especially in women of childbearing age.

How should Jenny's anaemia be assessed clinically?

Jenny should have a history taken and a physical examination performed looking for clues to the cause of her anaemia.

Mild degrees of anaemia are difficult to assess clinically. The palmar creases become pale as anaemia progresses. The conjunctival membranes become pale and

Haematology: Clinical Cases Uncovered. By S. McCann, R. Foà,
O. Smith and E. Conneally. Published 2009 by Blackwell
Publishing, ISBN: 978-1-4051-8322-2

the sides of the mouth may become sore. In some patients who do not seek medical attention, the anaemia may become very severe and you may see nail changes (spooning of the nails, koilonychia) or there may be dysphagia caused by a pharyngeal web.

Some patients who have chronic and severe anaemia develop a craving for potato chips or other substances such as crushed ice or clay in young children (pica).

> **KEY POINT**
>
> It is common for patients to have no physical signs of anaemia other than some degree of pallor.

What should be done next?

A full blood count (Table 4) and ask for a blood film (Fig. 14).

What do these results indicate?

Red cells that are small (low MCV) and pale (low MCH) commonly reflect iron deficiency.

> **KEY POINT**
>
> A deficiency of iron leads to a reduction of haem in the red cells and as a result the rate of synthesis of globin chains is decreased. The platelet count is elevated in patients with iron deficiency even in the absence of blood loss.

What is the differential diagnosis when red cells are small and pale?

The differential diagnosis should include a congenital deficiency in globin chain synthesis (thalassaemia syndromes), the anaemia of chronic disease, sideroblastic anaemia because of vitamin B_6 deficiency (pyridoxine). Vitamin A and C deficiency may be seen in severe nutritional deficiency.

Table 4 Results of full blood count and blood film.

	Patient results	Normal range (female)
Hb	8.0 g/dL	11.5–16.4 g/dL
MCV	62 fL	83–99 fL (μm^3)
MCH	19.0 pg/cell	26.7–32.5 pg/cell
MCHC	30 g/dL	30.8–34.6 g/dL
WBC	5.3×10^9/L	4.0–11.0×10^9/L (10^3/μL)
Platelets	550×10^9/L	140–450×10^9/L (10^3/μL)

Hb, haemoglobin; MCH, mean corpuscular haemoglobin; MCHC, mean corpuscular haemoglobin concentration; MCV, mean corpuscular volume; WBC, white blood cell count.

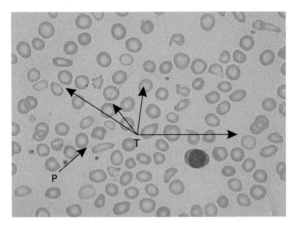

Figure 14 Blood film showing red blood cells that are small and pale. Pencil-shaped cells (P) and target cells (T) are also present.

What reasons would you give, for and against, the aforementioned diagnoses?

The inherited disorders of haemoglobin synthesis, thalassaemias, are uncommon in Caucasians but are seen in people from the Mediterranean, Middle East and South-East Asia. The symptoms and blood findings in patients with thalassaemia will depend on the degree of severity of the genetic defect. People with mild forms of thalassaemia may also have iron deficiency. Some of the tests for thalassaemia may be partially masked by concomitant iron deficiency. The anaemia of 'chronic disease' is seen in patients with chronic inflammatory disorders or cancer. It does not seem likely this patient has cancer or a chronic inflammatory disease because of her age and lack of any symptoms suggestive of the above.

What other investigations will help to confirm your suspected diagnosis?

In most instances, measurement of the serum ferritin level will give you an accurate reflection of the iron status. Serum ferritin is low in iron deficiency and normal in thalassaemia, and normal or raised in the anaemia of chronic disease.

Normal range for serum ferritin is 20–300 μg/L (ng/mL). Serum ferritin is an 'acute phase reactant' and therefore can be elevated in chronic inflammatory conditions or cancer (anaemia of chronic disease) or liver disease.

At what level of serum ferritin would you be prepared to accept iron deficiency as the probable diagnosis?

A level of <10 μg/L (ng/mL).

It is likely that Jenny has iron deficiency. What is the next step?

Take a detailed dietary history from Jenny and assess her iron intake.

In order to try to uncover the underlying cause of her iron deficiency consideration must be given to the way the body handles iron. The daily intake and the daily requirements for iron are almost equal. Therefore anything that increases iron requirements or causes chronic iron loss, e.g. bleeding, will result in iron deficiency.

KEY POINTS

In healthy adults the majority of dietary iron is not absorbed. However, this can be increased in iron deficiency by 20–30%. Iron is absorbed from the proximal small bowel.

Most body iron is contained in circulating red blood cells. When red blood cells die in the reticuloendothelial system, the iron is reutilized for the synthesis of haemoglobin. After red blood cell death the iron in the macrophages is transferred to plasma transferrin and then to the maturing red blood cell precursors in the bone marrow, which have transferrin receptors. The amount of iron required on a daily basis to compensate for iron loss from shedding of enterocytes (the epithelial cells lining the gastrointestinal tract) into the gut and growth requirements is almost identical to iron availability from the diet. Therefore, any excess iron loss is easily converted into iron deficiency anaemia. Menstruating females are thus particularly prone to iron deficiency anaemia.

PART 2: CASES

What contribution is dietary deficiency likely to make to Jenny's iron deficiency?

It would be very unlikely that a dietary deficiency of iron would be the sole cause of Jenny's anaemia.

Jenny has a full-time job, has a steady relationship and appears well nourished. She eats meat and vegetables regularly. People who are strict vegetarians are at risk of dietary iron deficiency especially during the teenage growth spurt. Poverty may be a contributory factor to dietary iron deficiency.

Normally, iron is absorbed into the enterocytes via a 'transporter' called DMT-1. The synthesis of DMT-1 reflects the ferritin levels. In iron deficiency, when ferritin levels are low there is less iron in the enterocyte. This leads to an increase in the synthesis of DMT-1, which causes an increase in iron entering the enterocyte. Likewise, the levels of ferritin and transferrin receptor (TfR) are linked. In iron deficiency, ferritin is low and TfR increased. Thus, the synthesis of DMT-1 and TfR respond to physiological needs.

Hepsidin, a small peptide synthesized in the liver, is a product of the *HAMP* gene and is an important negative regulator of iron absorption. Hepsidin synthesis is markedly increased in the anaemia of chronic disease and 'blocks' the escape of iron from macrophages thereby limiting its availability to form haem.

> **KEY POINT**
>
> Iron deficiency is never a diagnosis on its own. You must always try to find the underlying cause. It is particularly important to exclude occult (hidden, asymptomatic) cancers of the bowel.

What common mechanism can cause a woman aged 35 to become iron deficient?

Excessive menstrual blood loss is the most likely cause of iron deficiency in this patient.

Blood loss in excess of 80 mL/month is called menorrhagia. In practice, it is very difficult to assess the menstrual blood loss accurately. Both doctor and patient are likely to overestimate or underestimate the loss. A detailed menstrual history should be taken. Young girls who are at the menarche may bleed excessively before a regular pattern of ovulation is established. Likewise, women who

are reaching the menopause commonly have excessive menstrual blood loss.

> **KEY POINT**
>
> If patients have a change in the pattern of any symptoms or signs they should be referred for investigation.

What other parts of the physical examination are important in trying to find the cause of iron deficiency?

Jenny should have a rectal examination and assessment for occult blood in the stool is mandatory.

> **KEY POINT**
>
> In a post-menopausal female or in a male, blood loss from the gut should be excluded. Peptic ulcer disease, reflux oesophagitis (Fig. 15) and cancer of the oesophagus, stomach or large bowel (Fig. 16) should be ruled out by endoscopy. The use of aspirin and non-steroidal anti-inflammatory drugs may cause gastritis and bleeding.

The test for occult blood was negative. Occult blood is detected by smearing a small amount of fresh stool on a special piece of cardboard impregnated by a wood resin called guaiac (Fig. 17). A few drops of developing reagent facilitate the oxidation of guaiac by haemoglobin

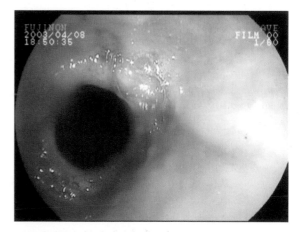

Figure 15 Endoscopic examination of the oesophagus showing oesophagitis and bleeding. This may cause retrosternal (behind the breast bone) pain or may be asymptomatic and present as iron deficiency.

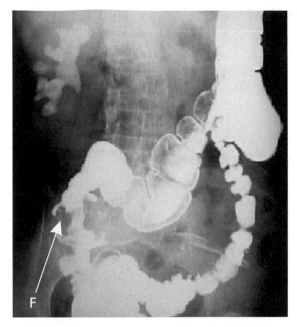

Figure 16 A barium enema, showing a filling defect in the caecum (F) caused by cancer. As the faeces are liquid in the caecum there may be no change in bowel habit and iron deficiency resulting from occult blood loss may be the presenting feature.

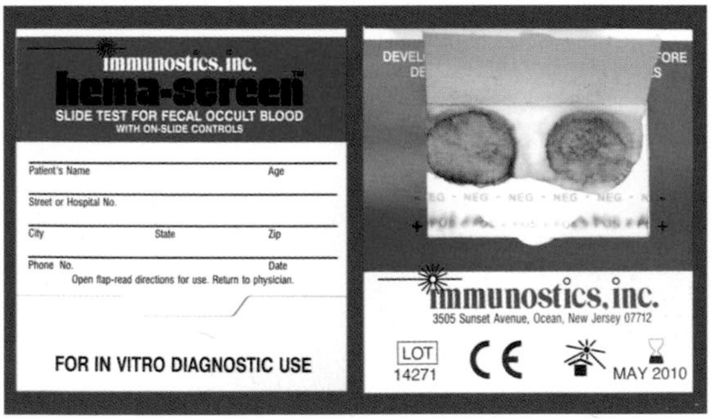

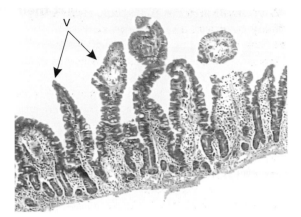

Figure 18 The normal pattern of the villi (V) in the small bowel.

guaiac-based test and is automated. It tests haemoglobin and no dietary restriction is required.

Blood loss from the bowel may be intermittent; therefore a single negative test for occult bleeding does not exclude gastrointestinal blood loss.

Screening of adults over 50 years for occult bleeding has been shown to increase the detection of curable colon cancer.

What bacterial infection can cause peptic ulceration and lead to iron deficiency anaemia?

Helicobacter pylori infection commonly causes peptic ulceration. It should be eradicated with antibiotics and proton pump inhibitors as it may lead to cancer.

What mechanisms are believed to cause iron deficiency in patients with *H. pylori* infection?

Possible pathogenic mechanisms involved in iron deficiency anaemia in patients with *H. pylori* infection include: occult blood loss secondary to chronic erosive gastritis, decreased iron absorption secondary to chronic gastritis causing hypochlorhydria or achlorhydria, increased iron uptake and use by bacteria. *H. pylori* eradication reverses iron deficiency in patients with asymptomatic gastritis and improves oral iron absorption.

What other disease mechanisms besides blood loss could lead to iron deficiency?

Patients with malabsorption because of coeliac disease (Figs 18 and 19) or severe dietary deficiency can present with iron deficiency.

Figure 17 A positive stool guaiac test for occult gastrointestinal bleeding.

and the colour turns blue. The test can be carried out by the doctor or the patient may post three samples of stool to the laboratory where the test is carried out. Eating large amounts of red meat, uncooked broccoli or horseradish within 3 days of the test can give a false positive result.

An immunodiagnostic test is also available for screening. This test is more sensitive and specific than the

How can the normal stature, lack of diarrhoea and anaemia be compatible with a diagnosis of coeliac disease?

Many adults with coeliac disease are of normal stature

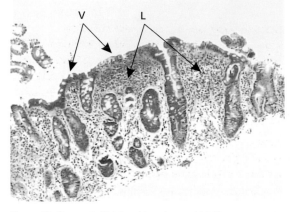

and have anaemia only. Failure of iron absorption may be augmented by excess loss of the enterocytes lining the small bowel. As folic acid is absorbed from the upper small bowel the patient may have concomitant folate deficiency.

If a diagnosis of coeliac disease is suspected, what further tests should be carried out?

Tissue transglutaminase antibodies (tGT) in the patient's serum are a reliable index of coeliac disease and if positive a duodenal or jejunal biopsy should be carried out to confirm the diagnosis.

Can you construct an algorithm for a patient with suspected iron deficiency?

Yes.

Figure 19 Flattened villi (V) and lymphocyte (L) infiltrate present in coeliac disease.

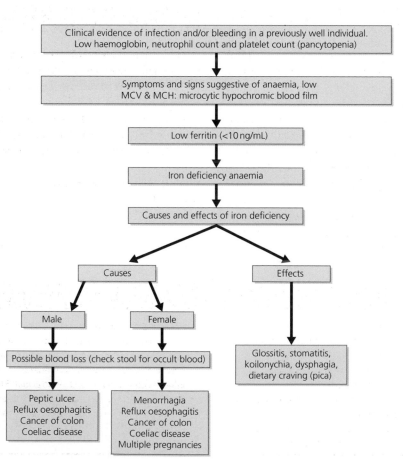

What are the principles of treatment?

Treat the underlying disease and give iron replacement.

How does the method of giving iron (intravenously or intramuscularly) influence the rate of Hb response?

The blood count will *not* recover more quickly with injections rather than tablets. In the majority of patients iron replacement should be undertaken while the underlying disease is being treated.

Oral iron therapy is almost always successful. Patients should remain on iron therapy for 6 months to ensure adequate replacement of iron stores. In rare circumstances, such as severe iron deficiency of pregnancy, intravenous iron may be used. Iron sucrose complex or low molecular weight iron supplements given intravenously are safe. The iron complex is taken up by the macrophages and the iron is subsequently released for incorporation into haemoglobin.

> ### KEY POINT
>
> If the patient does not respond (a rise in Hb of approximately 1 g/dL every 3 weeks) reconsider the diagnosis.

Outcome. Jenny had an upper gastrointestinal tract endoscopy and was found to have reflux oesophagitis and bleeding. This was believed to be the cause of her anaemia. She was advised to stop smoking and restrict her alcohol intake. She was given oral iron replacement for 6 months. She was given a course of proton pump inhibitors and advised to return to her family doctor in 2 months for a blood count. When she went to her family doctor her Hb was 11.5 g/dL and she was advised to take the iron tablets for a further 5 months to replenish her iron stores.

CASE REVIEW

A 35-year-old secretary presents with non-specific symptoms and very few physical signs. In an otherwise healthy young woman anaemia is high on the list of possible diagnoses.

Anaemia is confirmed by a simple blood test and judging by the red cell indices iron deficiency seems to be the most likely diagnosis. Menorrhagia is a common cause of iron deficiency and the history is often unhelpful. There is no definitive test and a change in bleeding patterns is sometimes a clue.

It is extremely important to rule out bleeding from the gastrointestinal tract and a rectal examination and test for faecal occult blood is mandatory. Remember carcinoma of the caecum. Cancer here may have no signs or symptoms other than iron deficiency anaemia, as the contents of the caecum are liquid.

Malabsorption brought about by coeliac disease is important to remember and many patients have *no* history of childhood diarrhoea and are commonly of normal stature.

In the vast majority of cases oral iron therapy will be successful.

KEY POINTS

- The differential diagnosis of hypochromic microcytic anaemia includes iron deficiency, anaemia of chronic disease and thalassaemia
- Iron deficiency can exist with mild forms of thalassaemia and make the diagnosis difficult
- It may be necessary to correct the iron deficiency before the diagnosis becomes obvious
- Serum ferritin is a good reflection of body iron stores but it is an acute phase reactant and will be elevated in inflammatory disorders and cancer. A level of <10 ng/mL is diagnostic of iron deficiency but higher levels may be seen when iron deficiency coexists with cancer (e.g. gastrointestinal cancer with bleeding) or with chronic inflammatory diseases such as rheumatoid arthritis
- The measurement of soluble transferrin receptors (sTfR) can help to differentiate between the anaemia of chronic disease and iron deficiency and is becoming widely available

Further reading

Andrews NC. Pathology of iron metabolism. In: Hoffman R, Benz Jr E, Shattil JS, *et al.* eds. *Hematology: Basic Principles and Practice*, 4th edn. Churchill Livingstone, 2005: 473–480.

Brittenham GM. Disorders of iron metabolism: iron deficiency and overload. In: Hoffman R, Benz Jr E, Shattil JS, *et al.* eds. *Hematology: Basic Principles and Practice*, 4th edn. Churchill Livingstone, 2005: 481–497.

Centre for Disease Control. Recommendations to prevent and control iron deficiency in the United States. *MMWR. Morbidity and Mortality Weekly Report* 1998; **47** (RR-3); 1.36.

Frazer DM, Anderson GA. Intestinal iron transport and its regulation. *American Journal of Physiology. Gastrointestinal and Liver Physiology* 2005; **289**: 631–635.

Hoffbrand AV, Moss PAH & Pettit JE. *Essential Haematology*, 5th edn. Blackwell Publishing, Oxford, 2006: 28–42.

Rockey DC. Occult gastrointestinal bleeding. *New England Journal of Medicine* 1999; **341**: 38–46.

www.mayoclinic.com/health/iron-deficiency-anemia/DS00323 Accessed on 7 March 2007.

Case 2 A 50-year-old tanned man with diabetes mellitus

Mr Peter Black, a 50-year-old engineer, went to his family doctor complaining of fatigue for at least a year, which was slowly increasing. He said he could only sleep for a few hours and woke early in the morning. He also complained of intermittent pain in the joints of his right hand.

What is the differential diagnosis?

The symptoms are fairly non-specific. Fatigue is always difficult to evaluate but could suggest depression. More information is needed regarding his sleeping pattern and activity levels during the day. He may be woken by pain and rheumatoid arthritis must be a possibility.

On further questioning Peter mentioned that he had gone to another doctor, with the same symptoms, 6 months previously. He had been under a lot of pressure at work and the first doctor felt that his symptoms were stress related. He had been prescribed sleeping tablets which he felt were not helping.

What further information is needed?

More information about his joint pain. A history of trauma, swelling or redness of the joints should be sought. You should also enquire about associated symptoms such as weight loss, fevers, night sweats or recent infections.

Peter revealed that he drank two gin and tonics in the evening and two glasses of wine with his dinner. He is a non-smoker.

On examination he is tanned and overweight. His liver is slightly enlarged. His second metacarpophalangeal joint is tender but not red or swollen.

Haematology: Clinical Cases Uncovered. By S. McCann, R. Foà, O. Smith and E. Conneally. Published 2009 by Blackwell Publishing, ISBN: 978-1-4051-8322-2

What else in his history may be contributing to his symptoms and signs?

His consumption of 28 units/week of alcohol. Although alcohol often helps people fall asleep, it also fragments the sleep pattern.

> **KEY POINT**
>
> Guidelines for sensible drinking suggest that a man should not drink more than 21 units/week (one glass of beer or wine or one spirit measure). Many people who abuse alcohol can continue to function at quite a high level.

What blood tests should be carried out and why?

A full blood count (Table 5) to see if the fatigue is caused by anaemia. A biochemistry profile and blood glucose (Table 6) to find the reason for the enlarged liver.

Mr Black returned to the surgery 2 weeks later. He was still fatigued despite stopping the sleeping tablets and reducing his alcohol intake. He mentioned that he was impotent, which he had been too embarrassed to mention initially.

How can the blood results be interpreted?

The elevated blood glucose suggests diabetes mellitus. His liver blood tests are also slightly abnormal. Although his haemoglobin is normal his red cells are slightly larger than normal (elevated MCV).

What other information might add to the interpretation of the blood tests?

The reticulocyte count, serum vitamin B_{12} and red cell folate level (Table 7).

Table 5 Results of the blood counts. The white cell differential was normal.

	Patient's results	Normal range (male)
Hb	16.5 g/dL	13.5–18.0 g/dL
MCV	100 fL	83–99 fL (μm³)
WBC	6.0 × 10⁹/L	4–11.0 × 10⁹/L (10³/μL)
Platelets	160 × 10⁹/L	140–450 × 10⁹/L (10³/μL)

Hb, haemoglobin; MCV, mean corpustular volume; WBC, white blood cell count.

Table 6 Results of the biochemical screen.

	Patient's results	Normal range
AST (SGOT)	60 IU/L	7–40 IU/L
Alkaline phosphatase	140 IU/L	40–120 IU/L
GGT	80 IU/L	10–55 IU/L
Random blood glucose	13.0 mmol/L	<11.1 mmol/L (<200 mg/dL)

AST, aspartate aminotransferase; GGT, gamma glutamyl transferase; SGOT, serum glutamic-oxaloacetic transaminase.

Table 7 Results of reticulocytes and vitamins.

	Patient's results	Normal range
Reticulocyte count	75 × 10⁹/L	50–100 × 10⁹/L (0.5–1.5%)
Serum B₁₂	600 ng/L	150–1000 ng/L (pg/mL)
Red cell folate	250 μg/L packed red cells	150–1000 μg/L (mg/mL)

How can these results be interpreted?

Large red cells (high MCV) could be reticulocytes caused by haemolysis. The vitamin levels are normal and therefore are not the cause of the high MCV. In liver disease lipid accumulates on the red cell membrane causing a macrocytosis.

In view of these findings what other information should be sought from the patient?

A detailed family history should be obtained because some types of liver disease are familial.

Mr Black said his father had diabetes mellitus but also had many other medical problems and had died from cirrhosis of the liver. This always surprised Peter, as his father was a non-drinker.

What should be done next?

He should be re-examined for evidence of complications of diabetes mellitus.

His blood pressure is normal. He has gynaecomastia (enlargement of the breast tissue; Fig. 20). His liver span is 18 cm (normal 12–15 cm; Fig. 21). There is no evidence of a peripheral neuropathy. Retinal examination is normal. Urinalysis shows glucose but no protein.

> **KEY POINT**
>
> As the blood glucose estimation was carried out on a random sample Mr Black was advised to have the test repeated when he was fasting (Table 8).

Based on the blood results is a diagnosis possible and if so what is it?

Diabetes mellitus, because of the combination of an elevated fasting blood glucose (9.0 mmol/L or greater) and

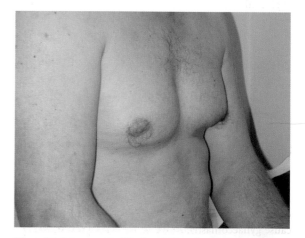

Figure 20 Enlargement of the breast tissue in a male, known as gynaecomastia.

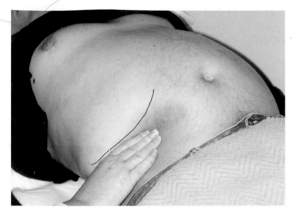

Figure 21 Palpation of an enlarged liver. The liver is not normally palpable. In this case, the lower edge is easily felt 3 cm below the coastal margin.

Table 8 Result of fasting blood glucose.

	Patient's results	Normal range
Fasting blood glucose	9 mmol/L	<7.0 mmol/L (<125 mg/dL)

glycosuria. The impotence could be related to a diabetic neuropathy but the gynaecomastia and arthritis are probably not related to the diabetes. The complications of diabetes and the follow-up care and diet should be explained.

The patient returned in 2 months' time. He had started an exercise programme, modified his diet and lost 5 kg (11.0 lb). However, he was still complaining of fatigue and a sore hand. The impotence had not improved.

On re-examination Peter is pigmented. His liver remains enlarged. He has loss of body hair and the gynaecomastia is more pronounced.

What causes gynaecomastia?

A number of drugs including spironolactone, cimetidine, imatinib, omeprazole and some antipsychotics cause gynaecomastia. Antiandrogens for prostate cancer and decreased clearance of oestrogen in liver disease are also causes. Tumours of the adrenals and testes are causes but in 25% of cases gyanaecomastia is idiopathic.

KEY POINT

Peter mentions that his cousin was recently diagnosed as having liver problems and was told his iron levels were too high.

What is the relevance of Mr Black's family history to his diagnosis?

It is probably very relevant. His cousin has liver disease and was told he had 'too much' iron in his blood. Mr Black's father also had liver disease and diabetes mellitus.

What is the differential diagnosis now?

To connect diabetes mellitus, liver disease, which appears to be familial, and the clinical findings a genetically inherited disorder in which the body absorbs more iron than is required for daily use must be suspected. The most likely unifying diagnosis is haemochromatosis.

Multiple blood transfusions and inherited diseases such as thalassaemia can lead to siderosis (iron deposition in organs) but are not relevant in this case. Likewise, myelodysplasia and congenital dyserythropoietic anaemias could cause siderosis but should not be considered here.

Because the body has no effective mechanism for excreting iron, other than bleeding, the clinical manifestations of haemochromatosis are much more common in men than women until after the menopause when monthly blood loss ceases.

How could a diagnosis of haemochromatosis be confirmed?

By measuring the serum ferritin and transferrin saturation (Table 9).

The serum ferritin concentration is a good measure of body iron stores but can be non-specifically elevated in inflammatory conditions. The serum transferrin saturation is the most sensitive and cost effective screening test.

There is no absolute abnormal value but transferrin saturations of >55–60% in a man or >45–50% in a woman are very suggestive of haemochromatosis.

PART 2: CASES

Table 9 Results of the iron studies.

	Patient's results	Normal range
Transferrin saturation	77%	<38%
Ferritin level	4250 µg/L	20–300 µg/L (mg/mL)

In 1996, mutations in the *HFE* gene were described and subsequently found in the majority of patients with hereditary haemochromatosis (HH). Two separate mutations have been described; the most common is the C282Y defect where a cysteine residue is replaced by a tyrosine residue. Ninety per cent of patients with HH are homozygous for the C282Y mutation. The second defect is H63D where aspartate replaces histidine. These gene mutations can be detected by a DNA-based test.

KEY POINT

The carrier rate for HH in people of northern European descent is 10–15% making it the most common genetic disorder in this population. There is a marked ethnic variation, with a very low frequency of C282Y in Asia.

Mutation analysis showed Mr Black was homozygous for the C282Y mutation (Fig. 22).

Figure 22 shows DNA, which has been amplified, from normal controls and homozygotes and heterozygotes for the *HFE* mutant alleles.

Dietary iron is transported into the enterocyte (cells lining the gut) by the divalent metal transporter DMT_1, among others. The amount of iron absorbed and transported to body stores is regulated by a number of proteins including HFE (*HFE* gene is on chromosome 6) found in enterocytes and liver cells. The precise mechanism whereby the mutated protein increases iron absorption is unknown but HFE works in conjunction with β_2-microglobulin.

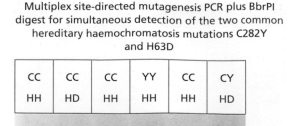

Multiplex site-directed mutagenesis PCR plus BbrPI digest for simultaneous detection of the two common hereditary haemochromatosis mutations C282Y and H63D

Figure 22 Polymerase chain reaction (PCR) is used to amplify normal and mutant DNA. Lanes 1, 3 and 5 are normal. Lane 2 is a heterozygote for the H63D mutation. Lane 4 is homozygous for the C282Y mutation (haemochromatosis) and lane 6 is a heterozygote for the two different mutations.

How might the diagnosis of hereditary haemochromatosis explain Mr Black's symptoms?

Increased absorption of dietary iron leads to organ dysfunction especially of the liver, heart, skin and pancreas. This would account for the skin pigmentation, diabetes and abnormal liver blood tests.

Disruption of hypothalamic–pituitary function because of iron deposition leads to hypogonadism, gynaecomastia and impotence.

Arthropathy, caused by iron deposition, is a common feature and occurs in 25–50% of patients. The joints of the hands, especially the second and third metacarpophalangeal joints, are usually the first joints involved.

How should Mr Black be treated?

Phlebotomy should be performed until his ferritin level falls below 50 µg/L (mg/mL) followed by life-long maintenance phlebotomy.

Mr Black should be referred to a hepatologist to be assessed for evidence of cirrhosis. Once cirrhosis develops, there is >200-fold increased risk of developing liver cancer. Phlebotomy is effective at improving a sense of well-being, normalizing the skin pigmentation and liver enzymes. The effect on arthralgia, diabetes and hypogonadism is more variable.

KEY POINT

Death is most commonly caused by cardiac and liver iron overload. If aggressive phlebotomy is initiated before end-organ damage occurs life expectancy, of patients with hereditary haemochromatosis, can be normal.

Mr Black says that he has three teenage children and wonders whether they should be tested?

They should be tested because phlebotomy, in affected individuals, will prevent organ damage resulting from iron excess.

KEY POINT

The disease is transmitted as an autosomal recessive condition; therefore, homozygotes (individuals with two mutant alleles) may have clinical manifestation of disease. Heterozygotes (individuals with a single mutant allele) are common and usually will not have evidence of disease. In HH, as in other genetic diseases there is incomplete penetrance, which means that although two people have the same mutation there is marked variability in the level of expression of the disease (Figs 23–25).

How practical is population-based screening for hereditary haemochromatosis?

Not practical. Variable penetrance means that not all patients with the mutations will develop evidence of iron

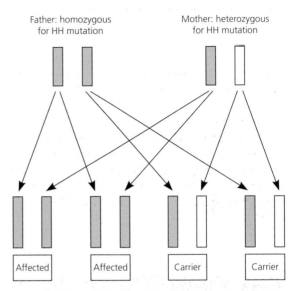

Figure 24 The possibilities for children of a homozygous father (haemochromatosis) and a heterozygous mother.

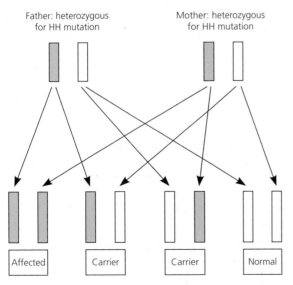

Figure 23 The possibilities for children of a heterozygous mother and father.

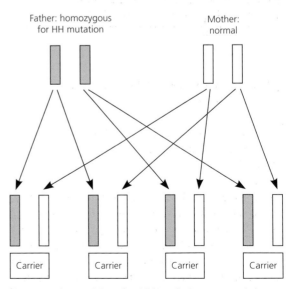

Figure 25 The possibilities for children of a homozygous father (haemochromatosis) and a 'normal' mother.

overload. Estimates suggest that it may be as low as 1%. There are also broader issues to bear in mind, such as the use of personal genetic information for the determination of life insurance policies. Up to 40% of individuals at risk of haemochromatosis could be identified by screening of first degree to third degree relatives of patients with iron overload.

Can you now construct an algorithm for a patient with pigmented skin and diabetes mellitus?

Yes.

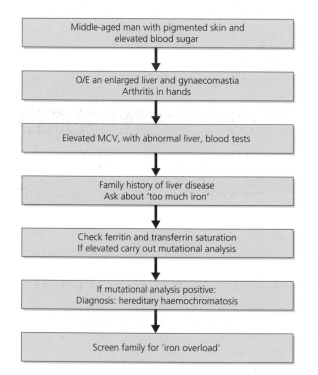

Middle-aged man with pigmented skin and elevated blood sugar

↓

O/E an enlarged liver and gynaecomastia
Arthritis in hands

↓

Elevated MCV, with abnormal liver, blood tests

↓

Family history of liver disease
Ask about 'too much iron'

↓

Check ferritin and transferrin saturation
If elevated carry out mutational analysis

↓

If mutational analysis positive:
Diagnosis: hereditary haemochromatosis

↓

Screen family for 'iron overload'

Outcome. Mr Black was started on weekly phlebotomy. He will be reviewed every 3 months and more blood removed to keep his ferritin level within the normal range.

His liver blood tests and MCV returned to normal. His blood sugar was controlled by diet. His impotence recovered but his hand remained painful.

CASE REVIEW

This patient had relatively non-specific symptoms. Because of this haemochromatosis is often not diagnosed at an early stage. Many of the complications of the disease are common primary disorders, e.g. diabetes mellitus, arthritis, hypopituitarism and cardiomyopathy and therefore the diagnosis of iron overload can be missed. Knowledge of the frequency of the disorder in the population you are treating is important.

The liver is the first organ to manifest signs of involvement and hepatomegaly is one of the most frequent clinical findings. Liver cancer is common in patients with haemochromatosis if they have cirrhosis; therefore early diagnosis and treatment are very important.

KEY POINTS

- Diabetes mellitus is a major issue and it is probable that iron deposition in the pancreas is an important factor although the precise pathobiology is unclear. Hypogonadism usually results from iron deposition in the pituitary gland
- Symptoms of haemochromatosis usually appear between 40 and 60 years. Men commonly present with symptoms of liver disease. Women are more likely to present with fatigue, arthralgia and hyperpigmentation
- Response of arthralgia to phlebotomy is variable

Further reading

Beutler E, Felitti VJ, Kosiol JA, Ho NJ, Gelbart T. Penetrance of 845G-A (C282Y) HFE in hereditary hemochromatosis mutation in the USA. *Lancet* 2002; **359**: 211–218.

British Committee for Standards in Haematology. Guidelines on diagnosis and therapy. Genetic Haemochromatosis. Darwin, 2000. www.bcshguidelines.com/pdf/chpt9B.pdf Accessed in Feb 2000.

Felitti VJ & Beutler E. New developments in hereditary hemochromatosis. *American Journal of the Medical Sciences* 1999; **318**: 257–268.

Hanson EH, Imperatore G, Burke W. HFE gene and hereditary hemochromatosis. *American Journal of Epidemiology* 2001; **154**: 193–206.

Olynyk JK, Cullen DJ, Aquilla S, Rossi E, Summerville L, Powell LW. A population-based study of the clinical expression of the hemochromatosis gene. *New England Journal of Medicine* 1999; **341**: 718–724.

Genetic disorder profile: hemochromatosis. Gene Gateway-Exploring genes and genetic disorders. National Digestive Diseases Information Clearing House (NDDIC), April 2007.

Case 3 A 65-year-old cranky woman with jaundice

Brian phoned the doctor's surgery. He said his mother, Ida, who was 65 years old, was unwell. She had been deteriorating over a period of 6 months, and recently was very cranky and her memory had worsened. She seemed short of breath when she came to answer the door and he thought her eyes looked a little yellow.

What might explain her symptoms?

Gradual deterioration and irritability could be caused by depression. Loss of memory for recent events tends to occur with advancing age. Alzheimer's disease, multiple 'small strokes' or a subdural haematoma could cause similar symptoms. Shortness of breath could be cardiac or respiratory in origin. However, there is nothing in the history to suggest respiratory disease.

Yellow sclera indicates jaundice. Painless jaundice in a woman of her age might suggest carcinoma of the pancreas, haemolysis or hepatitis.

I Brian was asked to bring his mother to the surgery.

What further information should be sought from the patient?

A full medical, family and social history. Previous illnesses such as gall bladder disease or jaundice should be enquired about. Sudden onset of shortness of breath in bed at night or on exertion and ankle swelling would suggest heart disease. Previous surgery, especially for cancer, would be very important as she may now have liver metastases. Ida's degree of memory deficit, using the Mini Mental State Examination (MMSE), should be assessed.

Haematology: Clinical Cases Uncovered. By S. McCann, R. Foà, O. Smith and E. Conneally. Published 2009 by Blackwell Publishing, ISBN: 978-1-4051-8322-2

Ida complained of a 'fuzzy feeling' in her feet and toes recently. She was normally a placid individual but he noticed she was definitely more irritable, for the last 6 months. Her husband had remarked that he noticed a slight 'yellowish tinge' to her eyes a few months ago. She is a non-smoker and non-drinker.

Ida has one sister, aged 70 years who has 'thyroid problems'.

> **KEY POINT**
>
> Unless specific questions are asked, patients may not reveal a previous diagnosis of cancer out of fear of a recurrence or forgetfulness.

What should be done next?

A complete physical examination.

She was slightly jaundiced and her skin had a lemon yellow tinge.

Her blood pressure was 130/85 mmHg. Jugular venous pressure (JVP) was raised and there was minimal pitting oedema in both ankles.

Deep tendon reflexes in her ankles and knees were absent. The plantar reflex was extensor (Babinski's sign). Appreciation of light touch was poor in both feet and legs. Her walk was slightly ataxic.

What is the differential diagnosis?

The differential diagnosis should include the possibility of diabetes mellitus but this would not account for her jaundice. An autoimmune disease or a vasculitis causing hepatitis and a neuropathy should also be considered. She could have underlying cancer with a paraneoplastic neuropathy but this would not explain her heart failure. Pernicious anaemia (an autoimmune disease) secondary to vitamin B_{12} deficiency could account for the shortness of breath, raised JVP and oedema, crankiness and neurological signs. The yellow sclerae are also compatible with this diagnosis as red cells are destroyed prematurely in the bone marrow.

Her sister could have autoimmune thyroid disease.

What investigations should be carried out?

A full blood count (Table 10), blood film (Figs 26 and 27), liver, bone and renal profile (Table 11), an ECG and a chest radiograph.

Table 10 Results of the full blood count.

	Patient's results	Normal range
Hb	7.0 g/dL	11.5–16.4 g/dL
MCV	112 fL	83–99 fL (μm³)
MCH	30 pg/cell	26.7–32.5 pg/cell
MCHC	32 g/dL	30.8–34.6 g/dL
RBC	2.2×10^{12}/L	$4.00–5.20 \times 10^{12}$/L (10^6/μL)
WBC	2.1×10^9/L	$4.0–11.0 \times 10^9$/L (10^3/μL)
Platelets	98×10^9/L	$150–450 \times 10^9$/L (10^3/μL)

Hb, haemoglobin; MCH, mean corpuscular haemoglobin: MCHC, mean corpuscular haemoglobin concentration; MCV, mean corpuscular volume; RBC, red blood cell count; WBC, white blood cell count.

The ECG showed a sinus tachycardia and the chest radiograph showed evidence of mild heart failure.

How can the laboratory and clinical findings be linked?

Ida is anaemic and jaundiced and the lactic dehydrogenase (LDH) is raised. These findings suggest premature destruction of red cells in the circulation (haemolysis) or in the bone marrow (ineffective erythropoiesis). The large size of the erythrocytes (MCV >99 fl) classifies this as a macrocytic anaemia and is compatible with a deficiency of vitamin B_{12} or folic acid. This degree of anaemia in a patient of this age could cause heart failure accounting for the oedema and raised JVP. The absence of deep tendon reflexes and the extensor plantar response suggest a combination of upper and lower

Table 11 Results of the biochemical test.

	Patient's results	Normal range
Bilirubin	28 μmol/L	0–17 μmol/L (0.3–1.1 mg/dL)
Lactic dehydrogenase	>5000 IU/L	230–450 IU/L
Potassium	2.8 mmol/L	3.5–5.0 mmol/L

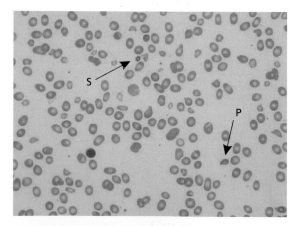

Figure 26 The blood film shows anisocytosis (variation in size; S) and poikilocytosis (variation in shape; P).

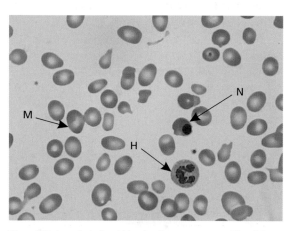

Figure 27 A nucleated red blood cell precursor normoblast (N), a hypersegmented granulocyte (H) and macrocytes (M), larger than normal red cells.

motor neurone lesions which is present in pernicious anaemia.

Other causes of a macrocytic anaemia include liver disease, aplastic anaemia or haemolysis.

Cancer must be considered in a patient of Ida's age and pancreatic cancer or liver metastases could account for the jaundice and the raised LDH. However, the anaemia would usually be normochromic or hypochromic secondary to blood loss.

KEY POINT

LDH is a ubiquitous enzyme present in all nucleated cells. Elevated levels are found in many cancers secondary to cell death. The highest levels are seen when red cells are destroyed prematurely in the bone marrow.

What blood test might help to clarify if the problem is related to haemolysis or ineffective erythropoiesis?

A reticulocyte count (Table 12).

Reticulocytes are present in the blood in small numbers. They mature into erythrocytes after about 2 days. A 'stressed' bone marrow can increase the number of red cells produced and this is manifest by an increase in the number of circulating reticulocytes in the blood.

The reticulocyte count is low in Ida's case, suggesting ineffective erythropoiesis. The reticulocyte count reflects the ability of the bone marrow to respond to anaemia. A high reticulocyte count is expected if haemolysis is occurring and a low reticulocyte count would be expected if there is ineffective erythropoiesis. The low white cell and platelet counts in this case suggest that there is ineffective haemopoiesis.

Table 12 Results of the reticulocyte count.

	Patient's result	Normal value
Reticulocyte count	25×10^9/L	$50–100 \times 10^9$/L (0.5–1.5%)

What essential 'building blocks' could become deficient and cause the laboratory and clinical findings?

A deficiency of vitamin B_{12} or folic acid could account for the symptoms and signs.

Vitamin B_{12} (cobalamins) and folic (pteroylglutamic) acid are both essential for DNA synthesis. A deficiency of either results in abnormal cell production in all body organs. The marrow is a rapidly proliferating organ. Consequently, vitamin B_{12} or folic acid deficiency will manifest themselves early in the peripheral blood. Once ingested, dietary vitamin B_{12} is attached to a glycoprotein, intrinsic factor (IF), which is secreted by the gastric parietal cells. The vitamin B_{12}–IF complex binds to a receptor in the terminal ileum where vitamin B_{12} is absorbed (Fig. 28) and transported in the portal circulation, bound to transcobalamin 2 (TC2). The normal diet contains up to 20 µg/day and the daily requirement is 1–2 µg. Therefore, the daily intake greatly exceeds requirements. The vitamin is found in animals only and is not affected by cooking. Body stores of vitamin B_{12} (in the liver) last about 4 years. It is a cofactor for methionine synthase, which methylates homocysteine producing methionine. Methyltetrahydrofolate is the methyl donor in this reaction. Methionine is converted into S-adenosylmethionine, which is involved in most of the methylation reactions in the body, e.g. the meth-

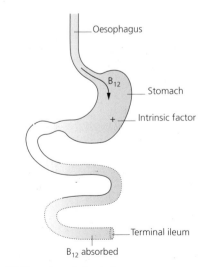

Figure 28 Absorption of vitamin B_{12}.

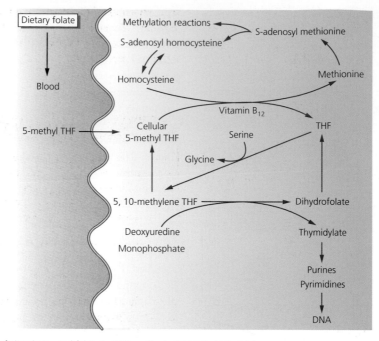

Figure 29 Interactions of vitamin B_{12} and folate in DNA synthesis. THF, tetrahydrofolate.

ylation of deoxyribonucleotides (DNA) and myelin (Fig. 29).

Folates consist of a number of compounds derived from pterolyglutamic (folic) acid and found in most foods including vegetables. They are absorbed through the duodenum and jejunum. An average diet contains about 200 μg, about 50% of which is absorbed. Daily requirements are approximately 100 μg and, in sharp contrast to vitamin B_{12}, body stores of folate last about 3 months. Folates can be destroyed by cooking.

Which vitamin is likely to be deficient in this patient?

Vitamin B_{12} deficiency is most likely because the symptoms are of gradual onset, she is elderly and she has neurological damage.

What should be done next?

Ida's serum B_{12}, red cell folate levels, parietal cell and IF antibodies should be measured (Table 13). Give her oral potassium replacement. Check for other autoantibodies.

Table 13 Results of vitamin and antibody levels.

	Patient's results	Normal range
Serum B_{12}	50 ng/L	150–1000 ng/L (pg/mL)
Red cell folate	200 μg/L packed red cells	150–1000 μg/L (pg/mL)
Intrinsic factor antibodies	Positive	
Parietal cell antibodies	Positive	

Start the patient on replacement therapy with oral folate, 5 mg/day and intramuscular vitamin B_{12} 1.0 mg every 3 days for 3 weeks. Check her serum potassium for the first few visits to make sure that the level returns to normal. A bone marrow examination could be carried out at this stage but it is not absolutely necessary (Fig. 30).

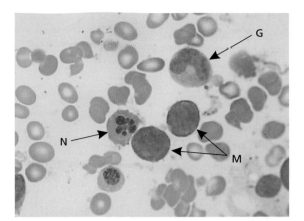

Figure 30 A bone marrow showing megaloblastic (M) red cell precursors. The maturation of the nucleus is out of synchrony with the cytoplasm and nuclear fragmentation is present (N). G, giant metamyelocyte.

in a worsening of the demyelination, which may be irreversible. Therefore all patients should receive both vitamin B_{12} and folate replacement until the diagnosis becomes clear.

> **KEY POINT**
>
> Treatment of vitamin B_{12} deficiency often results in a rapid improvement in the mental state of the patient. In long-standing disease the spinal cord abnormalities are not reversible and that is why early diagnosis is so important.
> Treatment with folate may precipitate neurological problems.

> **KEY POINT**
>
> A deficiency of vitamin B_{12} or folate will cause distinctive changes in the bone marrow. The difficulty in DNA synthesis leads to the premature cell death and ineffective erythropoiesis. Nuclear maturation is delayed, resulting in a distinct appearance known as megaloblastic change.

Ida has a low vitamin B_{12} level with positive IF and parietal cell antibodies.

Now what is your differential diagnosis?

Ida has pernicious anaemia, an autoimmune disease.

Why should she be given folate and vitamin B_{12} replacement?

A deficiency of vitamin B_{12} leads to demyelination of the brain and spinal cord (subacute combined degeneration). This does not occur with folate deficiency. The clinical manifestations are confusion and memory loss together with a combination of signs in the lower limbs reflecting demyelination of the posterior and lateral columns of the spinal cord, a syndrome known as subacute combined degeneration.

Giving folate alone to an individual who has vitamin B_{12} deficiency may correct the blood findings but result

What is the connection between the low serum potassium level and the vitamin B_{12} deficiency?

The abnormal DNA synthesis affects the cells lining the renal tubules leading to a potassium wasting syndrome. This results in low serum potassium.

> **KEY POINT**
>
> Treatment should begin with intramuscular vitamin B_{12} continued for life. When the patient has responded a change to oral vitamin B_{12} is possible, but compliance is a potential problem and the patient should be seen annually. When effective treatment with vitamin B_{12} is given there will be a sudden burst of activity in the marrow with many new healthy cells being formed and the serum potassium may fall further leading to sudden death. Therefore it is important to give early potassium replacement and to monitor potassium levels in the first week of treatment.

What else in the history is relevant to the diagnosis of an autoimmune disease?

A family history of other autoimmune disease such as thyroid disease in her sister. There is an increased incidence of Addison's disease (hypoadrenalism) in first degree relatives of patients with autoimmune B_{12} deficiency (pernicious anaemia).

What haematological response is expected from vitamin B_{12} replacement?

The reticulocyte count begins to increase within 2–3 days reflecting the new healthy red cells being released from the marrow into the blood. The red cell count will increase within 1–2 weeks and the MCV will return to normal over 4–6 weeks.

What mechanisms might make an individual vitamin B_{12} deficient?

In this age group pernicious anaemia is the most common cause of vitamin B_{12} deficiency; however, other causes include: partial or total gastrectomy, Crohn's disease (with or without ileal resection), blind loop syndromes, tropical sprue and fish tapeworm.

What is the Schilling test?

The Schilling test uses radioactive isotopes to measure the excretion of vitamin B_{12} in the urine. It can differentiate between pernicious anaemia and other mechanisms of vitamin B_{12} deficiency. The use of radioactive-based tests has become much less frequent with the development of reliable serum assays.

> **KEY POINT**
>
> It is increasingly being recognized that vegans and people in 'old peoples' homes' where dietary protein may be minimal may develop vitamin B_{12} deficiency. It can also be seen occasionally in young people.

> **KEY POINT**
>
> Deficiencies of vitamin B_{12} or folate may be significant contributors to vascular dementia and Alzheimer's disease because of the elevated levels of homocysteine (Fig. 29).

Can you now construct an algorithm to investigate a patient with pancytopenia?

Yes.

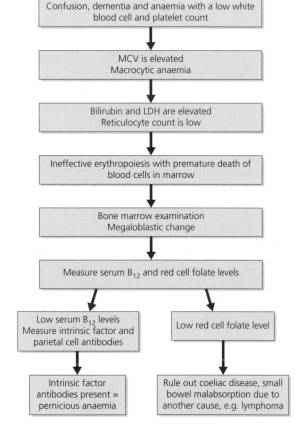

A 30-year-old woman was referred from the infertility clinic because she had a raised MCV (macrocytosis). Serum B_{12} was low and IF antibodies were detected. Within 2 months of replacement therapy she became pregnant.

Outcome. Ida responded well to vitamin B_{12} replacement with a return of her blood and biochemical tests to normal after 5 weeks. Her mental state improved even more quickly and she enjoyed seeing her grandchildren again. The doctor advised her to take her vitamin B_{12} indefinitely and to come for 6-monthly blood counts and medical checks.

CASE REVIEW

This 65-year-old woman had a history of deteriorating memory. The possibilities initially included CNS disease, or perhaps cancer. On examination she was jaundiced and had heart failure. The diagnosis still was not clear but the presence of Babinsky's sign together with the history of mental deterioration and jaundice made the possibility of cancer more real. The haematological investigations proved very informative. The presence of macrocytosis and pancytopaenia suggested an underlying megaloblastic change in her marrow. The very high LDH, together with the above haematological findings, is almost diagnostic of ineffective erythropoiesis secondary to megaloblastosis. Although high levels of LDH can be found in cancer, the levels rarely approximate those found in pernicious anaemia. The low reticulocyte count confirms the inability of the marrow to mount a response to the anaemia.

Although there are a number of causes of megaloblastic change in a woman of her age, with her deteriorating memory and Babinsky's sign a diagnosis of pernicious anaemia is almost certain. The low serum vitamin B_{12} level and the positive intrinsic factor antibodies confirm the diagnosis. The rapid response to treatment, especially the improvement in her mental state, is also confirmative of the underlying diagnosis.

KEY POINTS

- Vitamin B_{12} deficiency causes megaloblastic change because of an interference with DNA synthesis (Fig. 29)
- All body tissues are affected (e.g. epithelial changes, potassium loss from the kidneys) but the disorder is 'haematological' because the bone marrow is such a rapidly proliferating organ and therefore the changes are seen early in the peripheral blood
- CNS damage takes the form of demyelination of the dorsal and lateral columns of the spinal cord and is probably caused by defective methylation of myelin
- Incorrect diagnosis and treatment of vitamin B_{12} deficiency with folic acid may precipitate a sudden worsening of the CNS symptoms and signs

Further reading

Asok CA. Megaloblastic anemias. In: Hoffman R, Benz EJ Jr, Shattil SJ, Furie B, Cohen HJ, Silverstein LE, *et al.* eds. *Hematology: Basic Principles and Practice*, 4th edn. Churchill Livingstone, 2005: 446–485.

Hoffbrand AV, Moss PAH & Pettit JE. *Essential Haematology*, 5th edn. Blackwell Science, Oxford, 2006: 44–57.

Hvas AM, Nexo E. Diagnosis and treatment of vitamin B_{12} deficiency: an update. *Haematologica* 2006; **91**: 1506–1512.

Weir DG, Scott JM. Brain function in the elderly: role of vitamin B_{12} and folate. *British Medical Bulletin* 1999; **55**: 669–682.

Wickramsinghe SN, Guest Editor. *Balliere's Clinical Haematology, International Practice and Research*, Vol. 8; No 3. Balliere Tindall, 1995.

PART 2: CASES

Case 4 A 25-year-old man with weight loss and diarrhoea

Brian Jones, a 25-year-old bus driver, went to the company doctor in April because he noticed that he was losing weight and had diarrhoea. He admitted that he had to tighten his belt by two holes. He did not wear a tie every day but definitely thought that his collar was a little looser.

How would you evaluate his signs and symptoms?

Weight loss can be difficult to estimate, as many people do not keep an accurate account of their weight. The fact that he tightened his belt and said that his collar felt loose suggests significant weight loss. The duration of the diarrhoea, its frequency and colour are also important.

Ask about the presence of blood and mucus in the stool or if the stool is pale-coloured with a foul smell.

He said he had been feeling unwell and noticed the altered bowel habit since Christmas. He was unsure of the colour and did not think the stool was particularly foul-smelling.

What is your differential diagnosis?

'Irritable bowel syndrome' typically occurs in young adults. It is often associated with 'stress' but not with significant weight loss. Blood and mucus could indicate chronic inflammatory bowel disease (ulcerative colitis or Crohn's disease). Diverticular disease may present with abdominal pain, fever and change of bowel habit but would be unusual in a young patient. Bowel cancer is a possibility but is usually seen in older patients. A malignant lymphoma may occur in this age group and there may or may not be a history of coeliac disease. Coeliac disease may present for the first time, in adults of any age, with a history of diarrhoea.

Haematology: Clinical Cases Uncovered. By S. McCann, R. Foà, O. Smith and E. Conneally. Published 2009 by Blackwell Publishing, ISBN: 978-1-4051-8322-2

What would you do next?

Take a social and family history.

Brian was never ill before. He smokes 20 cigarettes per day and only drinks at weekends when he has a 'few pints' on a Friday and Saturday night. He has one brother and one sister, both older than him and they are both very well. His parents are well and he does not know much about his extended family. Brian lives at home with his parents and eats his main meal with them every day.

What should be done next?

A physical examination. On physical examination Brian was nervous with sweaty palms and a pulse of 100 beats/minute (normal 75–85 beats/minute). Weight loss was apparent because of his loosely fitting clothes. He had pale conjunctivae and palmar creases. His abdomen was soft but no masses or organomegaly were palpable.

What do the physical signs suggest?

He is clearly ill as he has a tachycardia and clinical evidence of weight loss. He appears to be anaemic.

What should be done next?

A full blood count (Table 14), blood film and biochemical screen (Table 15).

The blood film (Fig. 31) was reported as having oval macrocytes (larger than normal red cells and oval-shaped rather than the usual disc), and abnormally shaped cells (poikilocytes). The platelets were decreased in number.

Now what is your differential diagnosis?

Macrocytic anaemia with pancytopenia (reduced white cells and platelets) suggests an underlying megaloblastic change in the bone marrow. This could be caused by a vitamin deficiency such as vitamin B_{12} or folic acid. The

Table 14 Results of the blood count and the blood film.

	Patient's results	Normal range (male)
Hb	10.0 g/dL	13.5–18.0 g/dL
MCV	105 fL	83–99 fL (μm^3)
MCH	30 pg/cell	26.7–32.5 pg/cell
MCHC	32 g/dL	30.8–34.6 g/L
RBC	3.0×10^{12}/L	4.60–5.70×10^{12}/L (10^6/μL)
WBC	3.5×10^9/L	4.0–11.0×10^9/L (10^3/μL)
Platelets	120×10^9/L	140–450×10^9/L (10^3/μL)
Reticulocyte count	30×10^9/L	50–100×10^9/L (0.5–1.5%)

Hb, haemoglobin; MCH, mean corpuscular haemoglobin; MCHC, mean corpuscular haemoglobin concentration; MCV, mean corpuscular volume; RBC, red blood cell count; WBC, white blood cell count.

Table 15 Results of the biochemical screen.

	Patient's results	Normal range
Bilirubin	22 μmol/L	0–17 μmol/L (0.3–1.1 mg/dL)
Lactic dehydrogenase	3000 IU/L	230–450 IU/L

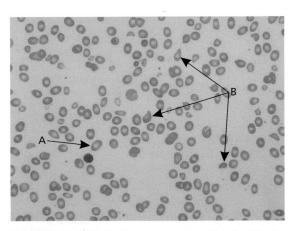

Figure 31 Blood film showing oval macrocytes (A) and poikilocytes (abnormally shaped red cells; B).

diarrhoea and weight loss suggest a malabsorption syndrome. Malabsorption of vitamin B_{12} could be secondary to gastric surgery but there is no history or scar, or disease of the terminal ileum such as Crohn's disease. Malabsorption of folic acid could be caused by a disease of the duodenum, jejunum or proximal small bowel such as coeliac disease or a lymphoma.

What test might help to explain the mechanism of the anaemia and the macrocytosis?

The reticulocyte count. A high reticulocyte count means the marrow is responding by making more red cells and a low reticulocyte count means that the marrow is incapable of responding.

KEY POINT

In this case the low reticulocyte count and the low red blood cell count (Table 14) suggest a production problem in the marrow. The biochemical screen also revealed some abnormalities (Table 15).

How can the biochemical findings be explained?

The bilirubin and lactic dehydrogenase (LDH) may come from prematurely destroyed red cells. Bilirubin is present in the unconjugated state before passing through the liver where it is conjugated. Thus, the unconjugated bilirubin will be elevated in haemolysis. However, in clinical practice, the total bilirubin is commonly measured. Thus, the biochemical profile enhances the suspicion of a 'production' problem in the marrow.

What mechanisms might cause the marrow to produce red cells that are too large?

Deficiencies of vitamin B_{12} or folate affect DNA synthesis in all dividing cells and because the bone marrow contains rapidly dividing cells, marrow production will be an early casualty. Abnormalities in the bone marrow are reflected in the white and red cell counts, which are readily available. Haemolysis or premature red cell destruction may lead to increased release of immature red cells into the circulation, which are larger than mature

Table 16 Results of serum, B_{12} and red cell folate.

	Patient's results	Normal range
Red cell folate	75 µg/L packed red cells	150–1000 µg/L (pg/mL)
Serum B_{12}	180 µg/L	150–1000 ng/L (pg/mL)
Serum ferritin	5.0 µg/L	20–300 µg/L (pg/mL)

erythrocytes. Chronic liver disease may result in large red cells because of lipid loading into the red cell membrane.

What should be done next?

Measure serum B_{12} and red cell folate levels (Table 16). Deficiencies of either of these vitamins can cause macrocytosis and pancytopenia.

How can these results be interpreted?

A low folate would suggest a malabsorption syndrome or a dietary deficiency. Folate deficiency resulting from dietary deficiency can be seen in young girls with severe reduction in food intake in an attempt to remain thin. In the severe disorder of anorexia nervosa multiple vitamin deficiencies occur. In severe poverty, times of war and food shortages folate deficiency can occur. Folate deficiency may also seen in multiple pregnancies as the developing fetuses compete for the vitamin.

Brian lives at home and eats with his parents so a dietary deficiency is unlikely.

If a dietary deficiency is unlikely, what diseases cause folate malabsorption?

Coeliac disease (secondary to sensitivity to gluten, a component of wheat) interferes with the absorption of folate by causing severe damage to the lining of the small bowel. Rapid turnover of the cells lining the small bowel (enterocytes), which are shed into the bowel lumen, also contributes to the low folate levels.

A childhood history of diarrhoea or a family history of malabsorption should increase your suspicion of coeliac disease. Ask him to find out if he had been investigated as a child for diarrhoea or 'failure to thrive' or if any of his family had been diagnosed with coeliac disease?

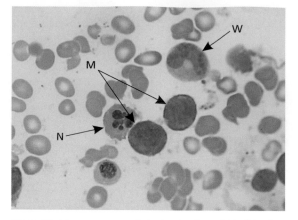

Figure 32 A bone marrow aspirate showing 'megaloblastic' red cell precursors (M) and 'giant' white cell precursors (W). The red cell precursors exhibit fragmented nuclei and delayed nuclear maturation (N).

KEY POINT

Many adults who present with coeliac disease *do not* have a history of childhood illness suggesting malabsorption.

What should be done next?

Refer the patient for specialist investigation because of the macrocytosis and pancytopenia.

The haematologist agreed that the presence of macrocytosis and pancytopenia warranted further investigation. He carried out a bone marrow aspirate, which revealed megaloblastic change (Figs 32–34).

In view of the diarrhoea and weight loss he also ordered a serum tissue transglutaminase (tTG) antibody test. The antibody level was elevated at 20 µg/mL (normal <5.0 µg/mL).

Now what is your differential diagnosis?

The most likely diagnosis is coeliac disease in view of the raised tTG antibodies and the megaloblastic changes in the bone marrow.

The combination of megaloblastosis and absent iron in the bone marrow suggests a combined folate and iron deficiency, which is seen in coeliac disease.

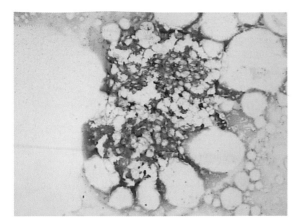

Figure 33 A bone marrow stained for iron, which is absent. In coeliac disease, there is a combination of iron and folate deficiency.

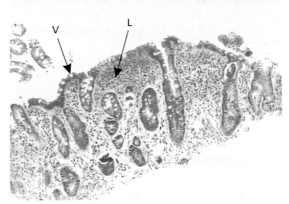

Figure 35 An endoscopic jejunal biopsy showing blunted villi (V) and an inflammatory infiltrate of lymphocytes (L) in a patient with coeliac disease.

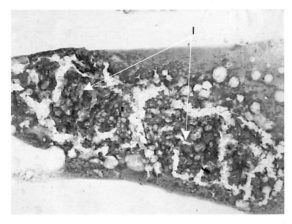

Figure 34 A megaloblastic bone marrow (folate deficiency). Iron is usually increased because of the ineffective erythropoiesis and increased rate of apoptosis. Iron is seen as a green stain (I).

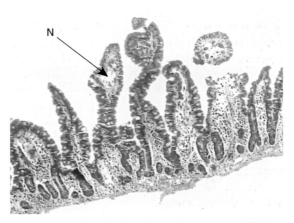

Figure 36 An endoscopic jejunal biopsy showing normal villi (N) and no lymphocytic infiltrate.

Tropical sprue, enteric (bowel) infections or lymphomas can present similarly but antibody levels would not be elevated. The presence of a small bowel lymphoma in a patient with pre-existing coeliac disease (undiagnosed) may cause confusion as the tTG may be elevated.

What other investigation would confirm your suspicion of coeliac disease?

A jejunal biopsy (Figs 35 and 36). There is some disagreement about the requirement for a jejunal biopsy but the majority of gastroenterologists carry out this procedure in order to secure the diagnosis and to observe the effect of treatment and patient compliance.

How can the megaloblastic changes in the marrow be explained?

A deficiency of folate leads to ineffective DNA synthesis.

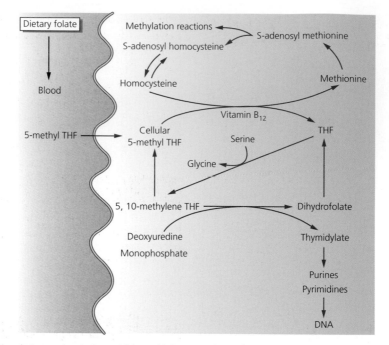

Figure 37 Interconnections between vitamin B_{12} and folate with homocysteine and DNA synthesis. THF, tetrahydrofolate.

KEY POINT

Deficiency of folate causes marrow damage because 5,10-methylene tetrahydrofolate (THF) is a coenzyme in the synthesis of thymidylate (which is required for pyrimidine and DNA synthesis) and of S-adenosylmethionine (which controls DNA production by its methylation; Fig. 37).

Folates are compounds derived from pteroylglutamic acid. The daily requirements are about $100\,\mu g$ and a 'normal' diet supplies about $150\,\mu g$/day. Folates are present in most green vegetables and liver but are partially destroyed by cooking. Folates are absorbed through the upper small bowel and body stores last for only 3–4 months, in complete contrast to vitamin B_{12} which last for years. All dietary folates are converted to methyl THF

by the small bowel. Folates are involved in many important biochemical reactions needing single carbon transfer.

KEY POINT

The appearance of the marrow together with the low blood counts (pancytopenia) reflects ineffective erythropoiesis, i.e. a production problem. In this case the iron stores are absent because of the malabsorption of iron, which also explains the low serum ferritin (Table 16).

Can you now construct an algorithm to help in the diagnosis of a patient with folate deficiency?

Yes.

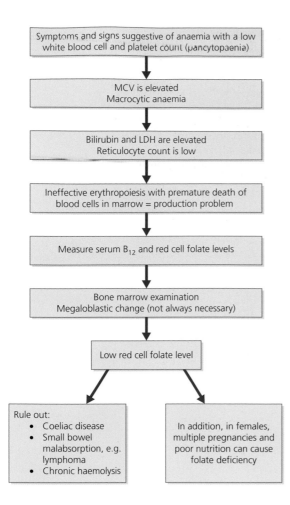

Outcome. A diagnosis of coeliac disease was made and Brian was placed on a gluten-free diet. He was given iron and folate supplements for 3 months. He was advised to stay on the diet for the rest of his life to minimize the risk of developing a lymphoma in his small bowel. His blood counts recovered, his bowel habit returned to normal and Brian returned to work 6 weeks later.

KEY POINT

Failure to adhere to the diet causes continual damage to the bowel and can result in the development of a lymphoma.

CASE REVIEW

A young man presents with weight loss and diarrhoea. He appears and feels ill. Malabsorption or cancer should be suspected although chronic infection is a possibility. He has no particular features of cancer and his blood tests show a pancytopenia and macrocytosis. This combination is very suggestive of a deficiency of vitamin B_{12} or folate. In vitamin B_{12} deficiency the iron content is increased because of ineffective erythropoiesis. There is no effective mechanism for the body to lose iron other than blood loss. A combination of megaloblastosis and absent iron indicates a problem of malabsorption in the jejunum and upper small bowel, as these are the sites of iron and folate absorption.

The combination of iron and folate deficiency in a young man with weight loss suggests coeliac disease.

This autoimmune disease is caused by sensitivity to a protein, prolamin, commonly known as gluten. Patients like this 25-year-old man may present for the first time in adult life. It is unclear why these patients do not present in childhood.

It is extremely important that an accurate diagnosis is made as in this case with serum anti-tTG antibodies and a jejunal biopsy. As well as being of diagnostic importance, compliance of a patient can be followed by repeated jejunal biopsies if necessary. Compliance to a gluten-free diet reduces the risk of developing a secondary lymphoma of the small bowel.

What other diseases are associated with folate deficiency?

A deficiency of folate in the mother at the time of conception increases the risk of neural tube defects in the fetus (spina bifida).

KEY POINT

Individuals who have the common mutation 5,10-methylene THF reductase (677C-T) have a greater risk of deficiency and giving birth to children with neural tube defects. Dietary supplementation with folic acid reduces the incidence of neural tube defects and is now recommended in all females contemplating pregnancy.

KEY POINTS

- The haematological combination of macrocytosis and pancytopenia together with weight loss in a young man suggests coeliac disease
- The serology and jejunal biopsy appearances are diagnostic
- Coeliac disease is much more common than was previously thought and may be as frequent as 1 in 300 in northern Europeans
- The aetiology is unknown but there is a disease link to certain tissue types (e.g. HLA DQ2)
- Patients with coeliac disease need to stay on a 'gluten-free' diet for life. Gluten is found in bread, biscuits, pizza, pasta and certain breakfast cereals
- Ground rice, corn flour, maize flour and soya flour are 'gluten-free'. Commercial gluten-free bread is available
- In long-standing malabsorption, vitamin D deficiency may occur leading to secondary hyperparathyroidism with a normal or elevated serum calcium, a low serum phosphate and a raised alkaline phosphatase

Further reading

Asok CA. Megaloblastic anemias. In: Hoffman R, Benz EJ Jr, Shattil SJ, Furie B, Cohen HJ, Silverstein LE, *et al.* eds. *Hematology: Basic Principles and Practice*, 4th edn. Churchill Livingstone, 2005: 519–556.

Farrell RJ & Kelly C. Coeliac sprue. *New England Journal of Medicine* 2002; **364**: 180–188.

Hoffbrand AV, Moss PAH & Pettit JE. *Essential Haematology*, 5th edn. Blackwell Science, Oxford, 2006: 44–57.

Hunt KA, Zhernakova A, Turner G, *et al.* Newly identified genetic risk variants for coeliac disease related to immune responses. *Nature Genetics* 2008; **40**: 395–402.

Kelly CP, Feighery CF, Gallagher RB & Weir DG. Diagnosis and treatment of gluten-sensitive enteropathy. *Advances in Internal Medicine* 1990; **35**: 341–363.

Molloy AM & Scott JM. Folates and prevention of disease. *Public Health Nutrition* 2001; **4**: 601–609.

A 30-year-old man with abdominal pain and jaundice

PART 2: CASES

Hans Neilsen, a 30-year-old male schoolteacher telephoned the surgery for an appointment. He said that he had been feeling very tired for the last 2 weeks and that his wife remarked that she thought he had yellow eyes. He also said that he had pain in his stomach, on and off, for a week.

What might be the problem?

His yellow eyes suggest that he is jaundiced and his fatigue is obviously significant as it was the first thing he mentioned. He might have hepatitis, gall stones or it could be a reaction to a medication. It is appropriate to give him an early appointment.

What general observations should be made?

Does he look ill or in distress with his pain? Has he lost weight? Is he jaundiced?

He looks well and is not distressed. He is not in pain and does not appear to have lost weight. His sclera are mildly icteric (jaundiced).

What questions should be asked initially?

Has the fatigue been getting worse? Is the abdominal pain becoming more severe, lasting longer or associated with any other symptoms such as nausea, vomiting or loss of appetite?

On closer questioning it was clear that fatigue had been a feature of this man's life. While at school he had not participated in contact sports because he always felt 'a little under the weather'. As far as he could remember there had

been at least two episodes of 'hepatitis' when he was 7 and 9 years old.

What is your differential diagnosis?

He could have had 'infective hepatitis' but the fact that it occurred twice should make you suspect another explanation. Other possibilities include: gall stones, pancreatic or liver cancer, drug-induced cholestasis, haemolysis with or without ineffective erythropoiesis, alcoholic hepatitis, autoimmune hepatitis and haemochromatosis.

Hepatitis is an infection of the liver. It is commonly caused by a virus and usually is a mild self-limiting illness. The most likely cause of infective hepatitis in a child would be hepatitis A. Other viruses that cause hepatitis include hepatitis B and C but these types of infection would be much less likely in an otherwise healthy child. Gall stones usually produce pain. Cancer would be unlikely in a man of his age and general well-being. He denies drug ingestion and excess alcohol use. Autoimmune hepatitis is much more common in women and haemochromatosis is a possibility but would not explain his childhood episodes of jaundice. Chronic haemolysis is certainly a possibility.

What should be done next?

A detailed medical, travel and drug history. Ask about any episodes of jaundice in family members.

Hans had always taken holidays in Europe and Australia. There were no other problems except an appendicectomy when he was 5 years old. He had one younger brother who was well. His mother was alive and well and his father had died 2 years ago of a 'heart attack'. He had no children. There was no family history of jaundice. He was not taking medication and denied use of illegal substances or recreational drugs.

Eye examination confirmed the presence of jaundice and his spleen was palpable 2 cm below his left costal margin.

Haematology: Clinical Cases Uncovered. By S. McCann, R. Foà, O. Smith and E. Conneally. Published 2009 by Blackwell Publishing, ISBN: 978-1-4051-8322-2

There was some tenderness in the right upper quadrant but his abdomen was soft.

Now what is your differential diagnosis?

He could have some form of congenital haemolytic anaemia (premature destruction of his red cells) with gall stones. This would account for the recurrent episodes of jaundice, enlarged spleen and abdominal pain.

Other causes of a large spleen, in a patient of this age, include Hodgkin's disease, non-Hodgkin's lymphoma, portal hypertension, chronic myeloid leukaemia and acquired forms of haemolytic anaemia. None of these diseases would be likely to cause the combination of symptoms and signs that this patient exhibits.

KEY POINT

Importantly, the patient looks and feels well, making an underlying malignancy unlikely.

What should be done next?

A full blood count, blood film, biochemical screen, urinalysis and blood pressure. A chest radiograph and an ultrasound examination of his abdomen should be ordered.

His blood pressure was 125/80 mmHg. His urine contained urobilinogen.

Hans should be advised to stay off work until the investigations are completed. The results of the investigations are shown in Tables 17 and 18 and Fig. 38.

How can the blood results be interpreted?

Hans is anaemic and has a high MCV (macrocytosis) and spherocytes. He could have haemolytic anaemia.

Other conditions that could cause anaemia and macrocytosis include vitamin B_{12} or folate deficiency or liver disease.

What test could help to confirm your suspicion of haemolysis?

A reticulocyte count, bilirubin and lactic dehydrogenase (Table 18).

Table 17 Results of the full blood count analysis.

	Patient's results	Normal range
Hb	12.5 g/dL	13.5–18.0 g/dL
MCV	103 fL	83–99 fL (μm^3)
MCH	30 pg/cell	27–32 pg/cell
MCHC	36 g/dL	30–36 g/dL
RBC	6.0×10^{12}/L	$4.5–6.5 \times 10^{12}$/L (10^6/μL)
WBC	10.5×10^9/L	$4.0–11.0 \times 10^9$/L (10^3/μL)

Hb, haemoglobin; MCH, mean corpuscular haemoglobin; MCHC, mean corpuscular haemoglobin concentration; MCV, mean corpuscular volume; RBC, red blood cell count; WBC, white blood cell count.

Table 18 Results of reticulocyte count and biochemical abnormalities.

	Patient's results	Normal range
Reticulocyte	130×10^9/L	$50–100 \times 10^9$/L (0.5–1.5%)
Bilirubin	25 μmol/L	0–17 μmol/L (0.3–1.1 mg/dL)
Lactic dehydrogenase	650 IU/L	230–450 IU/L

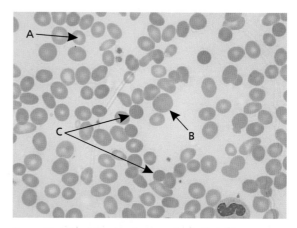

Figure 38 A blood film showing normal red cells with central pallor (A), polychromasia (grey–blue cells synthesizing haemoglobin (B) and spherocytes which are smaller and denser than normal red cells and have no central pallor (C).

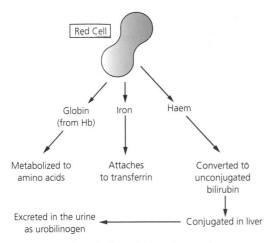

Figure 39 Normally, red cells are broken down in the reticuloendothelial system (liver, spleen and bone marrow) after 120 days in the circulation. The haem, which is converted to bilirubin, can cause jaundice and pigment gall stones.

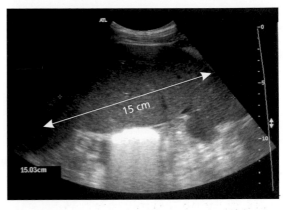

Figure 40 Ultrasound scan of the left upper quadrant of the abdomen. The dark grey area (under the arrow) represents the spleen, which is enlarged measuring 15 cm (normal 11–12 cm). This test uses sound waves to 'image' the internal organs without the use of radiation.

Now what is the likely diagnosis?

The elevated reticulocyte count suggests that the bone marrow is producing young red cells in response to the anaemia. These young red cells, reticulocytes, are larger than mature red cells, which explain the raised MCV. The elevated bilirubin and lactic dehydrogenase (LDH) and the urobilinogen in the urine are the result of red cell destruction (Fig. 39). The level of indirect (unconjugated) bilirubin is elevated in haemolysis. The spherocytes indicate a congenital or acquired membrane defect.

Hereditary spherocytosis (HS) is caused by an inherited deficiency or mutation of the red cell cytoskeleton, spectrin protein complex, membrane protein 4.1 or actin.

> **KEY POINT**
>
> In this case it is likely that the patient never had 'infective hepatitis' but instead had episodes of jaundice associated with haemolysis.

What should the patient and his wife be told?

Hans probably has a congenital disorder of his red cells, leading to their premature destruction. He should be referred to the next available outpatient haematology clinic, but this is not an emergency. The discomfort in his right upper quadrant is probably caused by gall stones and Hans might need to have his gallbladder removed.

What medication should he be offered and why?

Folic acid should be prescribed.

> **KEY POINT**
>
> Chronic haemolysis increases the requirement for folate, which is a major coenzyme in nucleic acid synthesis. Depletion of folate will inhibit the production of new red cells and the anaemia will become more marked.

What might suggest that the patient was becoming deficient in folic acid?

The reticulocyte count would be reduced and the anaemia would become more severe.

Hans was seen by a haematologist the following week. She confirmed the history and physical findings. The chest radiography was normal and the ultrasound of the abdomen (Fig. 40) confirmed an enlarged spleen.

What further tests should she order?

A direct antiglobulin test (Coombs' test).

This test detects the presence of autoantibody on the red blood cell surface (for a full explanation of the antiglobulin test see Case 6).

> The direct antiglobulin test was negative indicating that the patient did not have an acquired autoimmune haemolytic anaemia (AIHA, i.e. antibodies were not detected on his red cells).

What further test could explain the mechanism of haemolysis?

An osmotic fragility test (Figs 41 and 42), which measures the ability of red cells to resist osmotic shock.

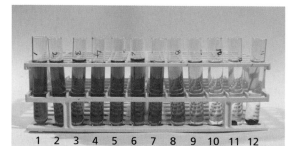

Figure 41 Osmotic fragility test measures the ability of red cells to resist osmotic shock (resistance to rupture when incubated in saline solutions). As normal red cells are bi-conave discs they are more resistant to rupture than spherocytes as they have a larger surface area to volume ratio. This is reflected by the amount of haemoglobin released when red cells are incubated in different solutions of saline and comparing normal with the patient's sample. Tube 12 contains normal saline and no haemolysis is expected. As the numbers go down to 1 the saline becomes hypotonic and there is a gradual increase in cell rupture and release of haemoglobin.

The result indicated that the patient's red cells were less resistant to osmotic shock than normal red cells, which was consistent with a diagnosis of a congenital disorder of the red cell 'cytoskeleton', hereditary spherocytosis.

KEY POINT

A bi-concave disc (normal red cell) will change its shape to a sphere when there is a reduction in the ratio of surface area to volume. There are two basic mechanisms to account for this shape change. Congenital disorders that lead to structural changes in the red blood cell 'cytoskeleton' will result in an abnormal spherical shape, the so-called 'hereditary spherocytosis syndrome'. Acquired autoimmune diseases, where antibodies become attached to the red blood cell membrane and are subsequently phagocytosed in the spleen, result in a loss of surface area and formation of a sphere (autoimmune haemolytic anaemia; AIHA; Case 6).

Two entirely different mechanisms can result in formation of spherocytes and premature red blood cell destruction.

What other investigation might help to confirm the diagnosis?

Flow cytometric analysis (see Part 1) will confirm the abnormal cytoskeletal membrane structure. Therefore, the patient has the hereditary spherocytosis syndrome. This syndrome is heterogeneous in terms of mode of inheritance, clinical severity and cytoskeletal lesion.

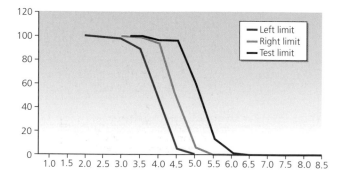

Figure 42 The black line is a measure of the degree of the patient's red cell rupture at the various concentrations of saline corresponding to tubes 1–12 (normal levels are between the purple and grey lines).

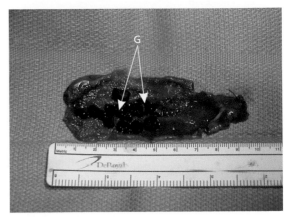

Figure 43 The gallbladder, removed at surgery, with multiple pigment stones.

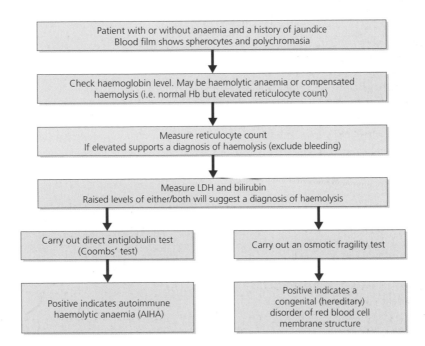

KEY POINT

The history of recurrent jaundice together with the evidence of haemolysis and a negative direct antiglobulin (Coombs') test is indicative of the hereditary spherocytosis syndrome.

What complications can occur in a patient with chronic haemolysis

Hans, like other patients with chronic haemolysis, may develop multiple small gall stones (Fig. 43), which may cause abdominal pain or obstruct the common bile duct.

These gall stones are the result of increased red cell destruction and increased haem metabolism to bilirubin. They are called pigment stones. If a small gall stone becomes impacted in the common bile duct, obstructive jaundice will occur and the elevation in bilirubin will be primarily direct (conjugated).

What other haematological complications can occur in patients with hereditary spherocytosis?

The so-called 'aplastic' crises. In this case the anaemia may be severe and is usually caused by infection of the red cell precursors with parvovirus B19. It usually occurs in children and is self-limiting.

Can you now construct an algorithm to investigate a patient with spherocytes in the blood?

Yes.

Patient with or without anaemia and a history of jaundice
Blood film shows spherocytes and polychromasia

Check haemoglobin level. May be haemolytic anaemia or compensated haemolysis (i.e. normal Hb but elevated reticulocyte count)

Measure reticulocyte count
If elevated supports a diagnosis of haemolysis (exclude bleeding)

Measure LDH and bilirubin
Raised levels of either/both will suggest a diagnosis of haemolysis

Carry out direct antiglobulin test (Coombs' test)

Carry out an osmotic fragility test

Positive indicates autoimmune haemolytic anaemia (AIHA)

Positive indicates a congenital (hereditary) disorder of red blood cell membrane structure

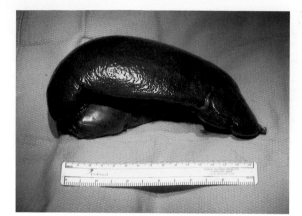

Figure 44 The enlarged spleen removed at surgery.

Outcome. Initially Hans was treated conservatively and given folic acid daily. His jaundice cleared but recurred 3 and 6 months later. He also had three episodes of right upper abdominal pain. Following vaccination against pneumococcus, Haemophilus influenza and meningococcus his gallbladder, because of symptomatic stones (Fig. 43) and spleen (because of recurrent anaemia) (Fig. 44) were removed and he was given life-long prophylaxis with penicillin.

KEY POINT

His reticulocyte count returned to normal within 3 days of surgery. Removal of the spleen will not correct the underlying red cell membrane defect but will allow the red cell lifespan to return towards normal. Splenectomy is not carried out on young children and should only be undertaken for recurrent anaemia and severe symptoms.

CASE REVIEW

A 30-year-old man presents with abdominal pain, fatigue and what appears on history to be jaundice. His story is fairly non-specific and he does not appear to be ill. On further questioning he has been fatigued all his life and has had a number of episodes which he calls 'hepatitis'. Although chronic hepatitis is a possibility the fact that he is not ill and does not admit to any history of medication, transfusion or recreational substances makes another diagnosis a possibility. If he has been fatigued since childhood a congenital disease is a possibility.

The most remarkable finding is splenomegaly. Again, this could be secondary to portal hypertension and chronic liver disease but there are no signs of chronic liver disease.

The blood count reveals mild anaemia and a high MCV. The platelet and white cell count are normal, therefore megaloblastosis is unlikely but the high MCV could reflect a high reticulocyte count. The blood film is very important, revealing spherocytes and polychromasia. The polychromasia reflects the high reticulocyte count as these cells are large and continue to synthesize haemoglobin, hence the colour. Spherocytes can be caused by an inherited membrane abnormality or a loss of membrane because of autoantibody formation and partial phagocytosis (Fig. 38). The direct antiglobulin test (Coombs' test) is negative, ruling out autoimmune haemolysis and indicating a congenital membrane defect as the cause of the spherocytosis.

Many patients with congenital membrane defects (hereditary spherocytosis) have a compensated haemolysis, i.e. almost normal haemoglobin but a high reticulocyte count. They may have the associated findings of pigment gall stones and icterus (jaundice).

Treatment consists of folic acid replacement for life and removal of the spleen and gallbladder if symptoms are a major problem and anaemia is severe.

> ## KEY POINTS
>
> - Chronic haemolysis presents with jaundice and blood counts show a high MCV
> - The high MCV is caused by a high reticulocyte count
> - Spherocytes in the blood film indicate either a membrane defect or autoantibody formation. The cause cannot be distinguished without the direct antiglobulin (Coombs') test result, as all spherocytes look the same
>
> - In clinical practice a negative direct antiglobulin test confirms a membrane defect as the cause of the spherocytes
> - Hereditary spherocytosis encompasses a large number of congenital defects of the spectrin–actin complex, which dictates red cell shape (the so-called cytoskeleton)
> - Treatment with splenectomy is indicated for severe disease and must be accompanied by life-long antibiotic prophylaxis and vaccination

Further reading

Bolton-Maggs PHB, Stevens PF, Dodd NJ, *et al.* Guidelines for the diagnosis and management of hereditary spherocytosis. *British Journal of Haematology* 2004; **126**: 455–474.

Delaunay J. Red cell membrane and erythropoiesis genetic defects. *Hematology Journal* 2003; **4**: 225–232.

Gallagher PG & Jarolim P. Red cell membrane disorders. In: Hoffman R, Benz EJ Jr, Shattil SJ, Furie B, Cohen HJ, Silberstein LE, *et al.* eds. *Hematology: Basic Principles and Practice*, 4th edn. Churchill Livingstone, 2005: 671–682.

Guideline for the diagnosis and management of hereditary spherocytosis. www.bcshguidelines.com Accessed in 2004.

Hoffbrand AV, Moss PAH & Pettit JE. *Essential Haematology*, 5th edn. Blackwell Science, 2006: 58–71.

Roper D & Layton M. Investigation of the hereditary haemolytic anaemias: membrane and enzyme abnormalities. In: Lewis SM, Bain BJ & Bates I, eds. *Dacie and Lewis' Practical Haematology*, 10th edn. Churchill Livingstone, 2006: 205–237.

Case 6   A 70-year-old man who was no longer able to take his dog for a walk

Hilliard Atler, a 70-year-old Caucasian man, went to his family doctor. He had a Jack Russell terrier for 10 years and usually walked him for 30–40 minutes in the evening. For the last few weeks he has noticed he was short of breath after about 10 minutes. This symptom had been getting worse to the point that he no longer feels he can walk his dog.

Can his symptoms be accounted for by his age or do they suggest an underlying illness?

A change in work or recreation patterns is always suggestive of disease.

What question(s) might define when the symptoms began? When were you last feeling well?

Were you well before . . . (use a well-known public holiday, e.g. Christmas, or national event)?

What associated symptoms should be enquired about?

Symptoms relating to the respiratory or cardiovascular systems. A history of previous episodes of shortness of breath, a cough productive of sputum or blood (haemoptysis), wheeze or chest tightness or discomfort on exertion. Symptoms such as ankle swelling or waking suddenly from sleep with shortness of breath suggest a cardiac cause.

Ask Hilliard if he has ever been treated for high blood pressure, angina, asthma or chronic bronchitis. Review his medications and his smoking habits.

Haematology: Clinical Cases Uncovered. By S. McCann, R. Foà, O. Smith and E. Conneally. Published 2009 by Blackwell Publishing, ISBN: 978-1-4051-8322-2

Hilliard said that he had been well all his life and 'never goes near a doctor'. He denies a history of the symptoms about which he has been questioned. He is a non-smoker.

What should be done next?

Take a full history, including a family and personal history of tuberculosis. A positive family history or contact with a person with tuberculosis could put him at risk. Travel to areas where unusual infections are present should be noted.

Hilliard has always taken holidays in Europe and has no known contact with tuberculosis.

What should be done next?

A full physical examination.

His blood pressure was 125/80 mmHg and his respiratory rate was 20/minute. His sclerae were jaundiced (icteric) and he was pale. His pulse was regular but slightly fast at 100 beats/minute. His heart size was normal and no murmurs were present but he had fine crackles at both his lung bases on inspiration. Hilliard had no lymphadenopathy but his spleen was palpable 3 cm below his left costal margin. He had bilateral pitting ankle oedema.

What is your differential diagnosis?

His pallor and jaundice suggest anaemia and liver disease, haemolysis or ineffective erythropoiesis (cells dying prematurely in the marrow). His rapid pulse, inspiratory crackles and ankle swelling suggest mild heart failure and his large spleen, an unexpected finding, suggests a haematological or infectious component to his symptoms.

What investigations should be carried out?

A full blood count, reticulocyte count (Table 19), blood film (Fig. 45) and biochemical screen should be performed.

Table 19 Results of the full blood count.

	Patient's results	Normal range (male)
Hb	5.8 g/dL	13.5–18.0 g/dL
MCV	121 fL	83.0–99.0 fL (μm^3)
WBC	7.9×10^9/L	$4.0–11.0 \times 10^9$/L (10^3/μL)
Platelets	450×10^9/L	$140–450 \times 10^9$/L (10^3/μL)
Red cell count	1.58×10^{12}/L	$4.60–5.70 \times 10^{12}$/L (10^6/mL)
Reticulocytes	320×10^9/L	$50–100 \times 10^9$/L (0.5–1.5%)

Hb, haemoglobin; MCV, mean corpuscular volume; WBC, white blood cell count.

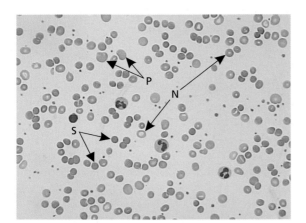

Figure 45 A blood film showing normal red cells (N), spherocytes (S) and polychromasia (P).

Red cells are biconcave discs and on blood film appear to have an area of central pallor. Most of the haemoglobin is around the edge of the cell and not in the middle, hence the appearance. Spherocytes are almost completely spherical but in a two-dimensional view will appear as a small dense cell without central pallor. The haemoglobin is equally distributed throughout the cell. The polychromasia or blue–grey colour of the red cells reflects the presence of ribosomes and haemoglobin synthesis. These young red cells are called reticulocytes. They are present in the peripheral blood in small numbers ($50–100 \times 10^9$/L). Premature removal of red cells from the circulation (from haemolysis or bleeding) will be reflected by an increase in the number of reticulocytes found in the peripheral blood as a compensatory measure.

How do the blood results alter your differential diagnosis?

The low haemoglobin means the patient is anaemic and the low red cell count suggests there are production problems in the marrow or that red cells have a shortened lifespan in the peripheral blood. The elevated MCV reflect the presence of an increased number of reticulocytes, which are large. This would indicate bleeding or haemolysis.

What is the significance of spherocytes in the blood?

Spherocytes indicate a congenital or acquired alteration in the surface area to volume ratio of the red cells.

Loss of red cell membrane alters the ratio of cell surface area to volume which results in the shape change. Red cells are normally very plastic and the biconcave shape facilitates reversible shape change as the cells traverse small blood vessels and the cords of the spleen. Spherocytes are inherently less plastic and have much more difficulty traversing apertures <8.0 μm in diameter.

By what mechanisms can normal red cell biconcave discs change into spherocytes?

Inherited abnormalities of red cell membrane, which interfere with the structure or function of the spectrin–actin complex (cytoskeleton), give rise to spherocytes, the so-called hereditary spherocytosis syndrome. Attachment of autoantibodies, with or without complement, to the red cell membrane results in phagocytosis of the attached antibody and/or complement by macrophages with subsequent loss of red cell membrane (Fig. 46).

> **KEY POINT**
>
> The mechanism of spherocyte formation cannot be ascertained from the blood film appearances.

What tests can differentiate the mechanism of spherocyte formation?

The direct antiglobulin test, also known as the Coombs' test (DCT).

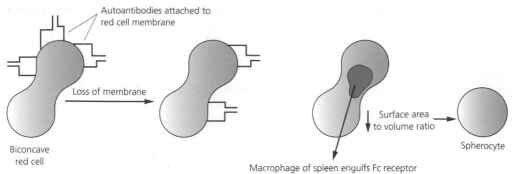

Figure 46 Diagram showing autoantibodies attached to the red cell membrane. Thus autoantibodies and endothelial cells in the spleen engulf some of the red cell membrane. Membrane is lost and a spherocyte is formed.

How does the DCT differentiate between the mechanisms?

The DCT detects the presence of autoantibodies (usually IgG) or complement (usually C3d) on the red cell membrane.

A reagent called the Coombs' reagent is used. This reagent is made by immunizing rabbits with human serum. The rabbit responds by making antibodies.

What components of serum does the rabbit make antibodies against?

IgG and complement.

How is the test performed?

Coombs' reagent is added to the red cells (Fig. 47) and the cells are centrifuged.

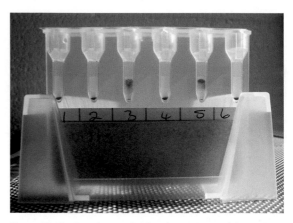

Figure 47 The Coombs' test (DCT). Tubes 1, 2, 4 and 6 contain normal red cells and the Coombs' reagent. After centrifugation in a gel phase, the red cells fall to the bottom. Tubes 3 and 5 contain red cells with IgG and complement on their surface. The cells clump together and appear to be suspended in the tube.

KEY POINT

If there are molecules of autoantibody (IgG or C3d) on the red cell membrane, the Coombs' reagent will bind to these molecules and bridges will be formed between the red cells. The result is that the red cells will clump together (agglutinate).

What other tests confirm a diagnosis of haemolysis?

Plasma bilirubin, haptoglobins and lactic dehydrogenase (LDH) (Table 20).

Table 20 Results of confirmatory tests of haemolysis.

	Patient's results	Normal range
Bilirubin	56 μmol/L	0–17 μmol/L (0.3–1.1 mg/dL)
Haptoglobins	Undetectable	0.45–2.05 g/L (mg/dL)
LDH	1404 IU/L	230–450 IU/L
DCT	Positive for IgG and C3d	

DCT, direct antiglobulin test (Coombs'); Ig, immunoglobulin; LDH, lactic dehydrogenase.

Now what is the diagnosis?

The raised plasma bilirubin (predominantly indirect) indicates destruction of red cells and causes the jaundice. Plasma haptoglobins are decreased or absent. The LDH is elevated as a result of red cell destruction. The DCT is positive, indicating autoantibody on the red cell surface.

Haptoglobin binds to haemoglobin, which has been released from the haemolysed red cell, and reticuloendothelial cells phagocytose the complex, thus haptoglobin disappears from the plasma. The diagnosis therefore is acquired autoimmune haemolytic anaemia (AIHA).

How should the patient be managed and why?

Mr Atler should be referred to a specialist. AIHA can be severe and life-threatening.

> **KEY POINT**
>
> The ability of the patient to withstand the effects of haemolysis will depend on the general state of health and any other illness that might be present such as heart disease.

What further tests will the specialist do?

Repeat the blood tests to see if the haemoglobin has fallen further. Carry out an ultrasound examination of the abdomen to assess the spleen size (Fig. 48).

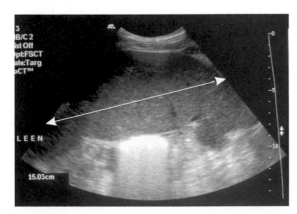

Figure 48 Ultrasound scan of the left upper quadrant of the abdomen demonstrating a large spleen indicated by the arrows.

Other diseases may be associated with haemolysis, e.g. systemic lupus erythematosus (SLE) or chronic lymphocytic leukaemia. Drugs such as penicillin, quinidine or methyldopa may cause AIHA.

What are the principles of treatment?

Give corticosteroids and monitor the response. Avoid red cell transfusion if possible.

Why should blood transfusion be avoided?

The antigens on the transfused red cells may stimulate further production of antibody in the recipient's plasma and increase the rate of haemolysis.

> **KEY POINT**
>
> Give folic acid orally. Patients who have haemolysis may become deficient in folic acid because of the excessive demand by the bone marrow to make new red cells leading to a worsening of the anaemia. A falling reticulocyte count with a further fall in the haemoglobin is suggestive of folate deficiency.

Which other types of autoantibodies can cause haemolysis?

Antibodies of the IgM class, so-called cold antibodies, can bind to the red cell surface and always bind complement.

The patient may experience acrocyanosis (purple discoloration of the extremities) in cold weather because of clumping of red cells in the circulation.

> **KEY POINT**
>
> Recently, patients with chronic haemolytic anaemia that fails to respond to corticosteroids have been successfully treated with anti-CD20 antibody (rituximab).

Can you construct an algorithm when you suspect haemolysis?

Yes.

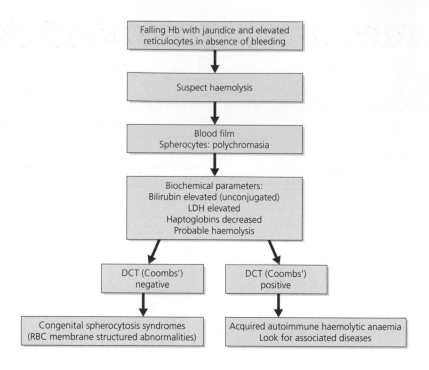

Outcome. Mr Atler was given oral corticosteroids and folic acid supplements. Antifungal prophylaxis and proton pump inhibitors were prescribed to counteract the major toxicities of corticosteroids and his blood glucose was monitored carefully. No underlying disease was detected and his haemoglobin returned to normal in 4 weeks.

CASE REVIEW

An elderly man complains of shortness of breath on exertion. He was icteric and had evidence of mild heart failure. The initial symptoms and signs could point to a number of diagnoses including cancer, ischaemic heart disease and liver disease. A critical finding is that of a large spleen. This raises the possibility of a haematological disorder and the icterus, pallor and heart failure suggest a form of anaemia.

The blood result is crucial, revealing severe anaemia with a high MCV and a reticulocytosis. This implies haemolysis and in a man of this age is likely to be acquired.

The blood film is diagnostic of haemolysis, revealing spherocytes and polychromasia. The direct antiglobulin test (Coombs' test) is positive. This clinches a diagnosis of autoimmune haemolytic anaemia and the loss of membrane accounts for the spherocytes in the blood film. The only way to distinguish spherocytes resulting from autoantibody formation from congenital membrane defect is by the direct antiglobulin test.

A diagnosis of acquired autoimmune haemolytic anaemia should always prompt a search for an underlying disease; however, as in this case, nothing else was discovered. Treatment is usually with corticosteroids and folic acid, but splenectomy may be required in resistant cases. Treatment of any underlying disease is indicated (e.g. chronic lymphocytic leukaemia; Case 11) and monoclonal antibodies to CD20 may be useful in switching off antibody production and reducing haemolysis.

KEY POINTS

- An elderly man presents with jaundice, evidence of heart failure and splenomegaly
- The blood findings suggest haemolytic anaemia
- Inspection of the blood film is crucial in revealing the diagnosis
- Spherocytes are present and the direct antiglobulin (Coombs') test is positive
- Although there may be an underlying disease many patients appear to have isolated autoimmune haemolysis
- The usual treatment is with corticosteroids but the precise mechanism of action is debated. It probably is a combination of uncoupling of antibody from the red cell membrane, Fc receptor blockade and a gradual reduction in antibody production by B lymphocytes

- Response to steroids is usually brisk but often incomplete. Treatment with immunosuppressive agents is commonly required in order to allow a reduction in the dosage of corticosteroids
- Patients may respond, have a prolonged disease-free period without treatment and then relapse for unknown reasons
- Folate deficiency, secondary to increased requirement of the marrow to produce 'new' erythrocytes, may compound the anaemia. This will inevitably be accompanied by a fall in the haemoglobin and the reticulocyte count

Further reading

Cunningham MJ, Silberstein LE. Autoimmune hemolytic anemia. In: Hoffman R, Benz EJ Jr, Shattil SJ, Furie B, Cohen HJ, Silberstein LE, *et al.* eds. *Hematology: Basic Principles and Practice*, 4th edn. Churchill Livingstone, 2005: 693–707.

Dacie J. *The Haemolytic Anaemias*, Vol. 4. *Secondary or Symptomatic Haemolytic Anaemias*, 3rd edn. Churchill Livingstone, 1995.

Hoffbrand AV, Moss PAH & Pettit JE. *Essential Haematology*, 5th edn. Blackwell Science, Oxford, 2006: 58–71.

Hoffman PC. *Immune Hemolytic Anemia.* asheducationbook. hematologylibrary.org/cgi/content/full/2006/1/13   Accessed in 2006.

Case 7 — A 35-year-old man with shortness of breath and anaemia

Ola Onyeabor, a 35-year-old computer analyst from Nigeria, presented to the accident and emergency department complaining of chest pain and shortness of breath for 48 hours. He was ill and distressed. His pulse rate was 120/ minute (normal 75–90/minute) and his blood pressure was 140/90 mmHg (normal 120/80 mmHg). He was tachypnoeic (breathing quickly) at a rate of 35/minute (normal 12–16/ minute). His oxygen saturation was 82% (normal >96%). He was jaundiced and his temperature was 38°C. He was given oxygen, pain relief with morphine and hydrated intravenously.

When he was more comfortable Ola said that he had been diagnosed as having sickle cell anaemia when he was a child. He could not remember much about his childhood illness but he had many admissions to hospital for 'painful crises' and had become dependent on opioid analgesics (narcotic pain-relieving drugs).

What investigations should be carried out immediately?

A full blood count (Table 21), a blood film (Fig. 49), a biochemical screen (Table 22) and a chest radiograph (Fig. 50).

| The blood film (Fig. 49) showed 'sickle' shaped red cells.

What is your interpretation of the blood findings in this clinical setting?

Ola is severely anaemic. The presence of abnormal 'sickle' shaped cells in the blood suggests sickle cell anaemia. The raised mean corpuscular haemoglobin concentration (MCHC) is caused by 'dehydration' of the red cells. The raised white cell count is probably a result of infection.

Haematology: Clinical Cases Uncovered. By S. McCann, R. Foà, O. Smith and E. Conneally. Published 2009 by Blackwell Publishing, ISBN: 978-1-4051-8322-2

Adults normally have haemoglobin A in their red cells. This haemoglobin is made up of two α and two β globin chains together with the 'haem' or iron-containing moiety.

KEY POINT

Haemoglobin is normally in solution within the red blood cell.

A large number of congenital diseases exist in which an abnormal gene encodes for an abnormal haemoglobin. If the amino acid 'substitution' results in an alteration in the function of the haemoglobin molecule then disease may occur. The most well-known disease is sickle cell disease, in which the substitution of a single amino acid, valine, for glutamic acid in the β chain results in reduced solubility of the haemoglobin molecule. When oxygen concentrations are reduced the haemoglobin polymerizes, i.e. comes out of solution and causes the red cell to become 'stiff' and change its shape into a 'sickle' cell. This leads to obstruction (vaso-occlusion) of blood vessels and infarction (death) of the distal tissue. It also results in premature destruction of red cells (haemolysis) contributing to anaemia.

What other blood tests might help to make a diagnosis?

The reticulocyte count and the biochemical screen (Table 22).

What do these tests suggest?

The raised reticulocyte count reflects the release of young red blood cells into the circulation and the raised lactic dehydrogenase (LDH) reflects red cell destruction. Both of these findings support a diagnosis of haemolysis.

Table 21 Results of the full blood count.

	Patient's results	Normal range (male)
Hb	6.70 g/dL	13.5–18.0 g/dL
WBC	18.7 × 10⁹/L	4.0–11.0 × 10⁹/L (10³/μL)
Platelets	343 × 10⁹/L	140–450 × 10⁹/L (10³/μL)
MCV	85.0 fL	83.0–99.0 fL (μm³)
MCHC	36.0 g/dL	30.8–34.6 g/dL
Red cell count	2.72 × 10¹²/L	4.60–5.70 × 10¹²/L (10⁶/μL)
Neutrophils	14.8 × 10⁹/L	2.0–7.5 × 10⁹/L (10³/μL)
Lymphocytes	2.0 × 10⁹/L	1.5–3.5 × 10⁹/L (10³/μL)

MCHC, mean corpuscular haemoglobin concentration; MCV, mean corpuscular volume; WBC, white blood cell count.

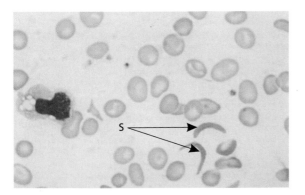

Figure 49 A blood film, showing 'sickle cells' (S).

Table 22 Results of the reticulocyte count and biochemical screen.

	Patient's results	Normal range
Reticulocyte count	275 × 10⁹/L	50–100 × 10⁹/L (0.5–1.5%)
Bilirubin	39 μmol/L	0–17 μmol/L (0.3–1.1 mg/dL)
Lactic dehydrogenase	524 IU/L	230–450 IU/L

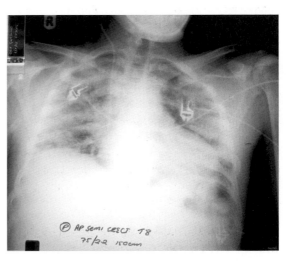

Figure 50 Chest radiograph showing bilateral pulmonary infiltrates.

He remained hypoxaemic with an oxygenation of 88% (normal >96%) and his chest radiograph was abnormal (Fig. 50).

How can the clinical and laboratory findings help to make a provisional diagnosis?

In Ola's case the most likely diagnosis is sickle cell disease and a 'chest syndrome' based upon new pulmonary infiltrates with fever, cough and chest pain.

It may be precipitated by an infection. The history, anaemia and abnormally shaped cells in the blood together with the evidence of haemolysis and the chest signs and symptoms all support the diagnosis.

What should be done next?

Ola should be admitted to a haematology ward.

What other treatment should be considered?

A blood transfusion might help because he is anaemic and his oxygen carrying capacity is compromised.

What special type of blood transfusion is sometimes considered for patients with sickle cell disease?

An exchange transfusion. This is carried out either manually by removing blood from the patient and replacing it with normal red cells or the use of a special apheresis machine. Exchange transfusion prevents sickle cells from contributing to vaso-occlusive events, reduces blood viscosity, adds oxygen carrying capacity and reduces haemolytic complications.

What are the indications for exchange transfusion and what is the desired result for the patient?

Exchange transfusion has been shown to be beneficial in children with acute vaso-occlusive stroke. A computed tomography (CT) examination should be performed prior to exchange to confirm the cause of the stroke. The haemoglobin should be raised to 10 g/dL and the Hb S level should be reduced to less than 30%. Exchange transfusion is also useful in the treatment of acute chest syndrome, severe cholestasis and multi-organ failure. Its value in treating priapism is unclear. However, it is considered prior to serious elective surgery, e.g. open heart or retinal surgery.

What are the potential problems associated with red cell transfusion in patients with sickle cell disease?

There are a number of potential problems:

1 Ola has had numerous previous hospitalizations and blood transfusions. Therefore he may have developed allo-antibodies. This will delay the transfusion, as compatible blood must be found.

2 The distribution of blood group antigens on the red cells of Nigerians is different from that found in Europeans, therefore it may be difficult to find compatible red cells for Ola (red cells with the same antigens as the patient's).

3 In some cases frozen red cells will be required from a blood bank from donors with similar red cell antigens to Ola.

4 Iron overload may be a problem for Ola unless he is treated with iron chelating agents.

What is the aim of the blood transfusion?

To increase the haemoglobin to approximately 10.0 g/dL, and therefore to decrease the level of abnormal haemoglobin (Hb S) in the circulation.

What will influence the spectrum of clinical problems experienced by individuals with sickle cell disease?

The clinical signs and symptoms depend on the ethnic origin of the individual (sickle cell disease is less severe in people from the Middle East than in West Africans).

The signs and symptoms will also vary because many patients have a second mutation in the haemoglobin molecule, which can protect against the tendency of the haemoglobin to 'sickle'.

The level of haemoglobin F (fetal haemoglobin) in the red blood cells in some patients is raised and this protects against 'sickling'. This may be because of a 'genetic adaptation'.

> ### KEY POINT
>
> Infection with malaria is common in areas where sickle cell disease is prevalent and elevated levels of haemoglobin F can protect red cells from damage caused by malaria parasites.

What else can influence the degree of 'sickling'?

The degree of 'sickling' will depend on whether the patient has inherited one or two abnormal (haemoglobin S) alleles.

If one normal and one haemoglobin S allele have been inherited the individual will be a heterozygote and have no signs and symptoms of sickle cell disease (sickle cell trait). If two abnormal haemoglobin S alleles are inherited the individual is a homozygote and will have all the problems associated with sickle cell disease.

> ### KEY POINT
>
> Under conditions of severe hypoxia some individuals with sickle trait may develop signs of 'sickling' in their red cells.

What tests should be performed to clarify the diagnosis and why these tests in particular?

A screening test called the 'sickledex' will identify haemoglobin S (Fig. 51). Electrophoresis of the haemoglobin will separate haemoglobin S from normal adult haemoglobin (Fig. 52).

This test will distinguish sickle cell trait (a heterozygote) from sickle cell disease (a homozygote). Figure 52

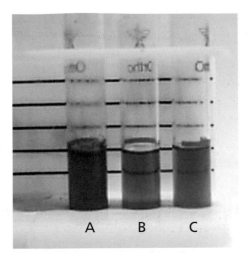

Figure 51 Turbidity caused by Hb S when a reducing agent is added to the blood. A contains Hb SS, B is normal and C contains Hb SA.

CAM alkaline pH

+

A

F

S,D+G

C,E+O

−

ACA acid pH

−

F

A,E,D+G

S

C

+

Figure 52 The separation of different haemoglobins by electrophoresis.

Table 23 Common haemoglobin variants.

	Homozygote EE	**Heterozygote AE**	**Country of origin**
Haemoglobin E*	Mild anaemia	Normal Hb level	SE Asia (up to 30% of population)
	MCV reduced	MCV slightly reduced	
	Target cells	Occasional target cells	
	20–30% Hb E		
	Homozygote CC	**Heterozygote AC**	**Country of origin**
Haemoglobin C	Chronic haemolysis and large spleen	Normal	West Africa
		Target cells	
	Mild anaemia		
	Reticulocytes increased		
	Target cells prominent		
Haemoglobin D†	DD	AD	
	Normal Hb level	Normal Hb level	NW India

MCV, mean corpuscular volume.

*Individuals with Hb E commonly coinherit thalassaemia.

†May be confused with Hb S on electrophoresis. Distinction is important for genetic counselling.

shows haemoglobin electrophoresis. Different haemoglobins can be separated depending on their charge and the pH of the gel. Note that in an alkaline pH Hb S and D are not separated (Table 23) whereas in an acid pH Hb A and Hb S are easily identified.

What other abnormal haemoglobins occur?

There are a number of mutant haemoglobins that reflect various amino acid substitutions in the Hb molecule (Table 23).

What other pathological mechanisms can contribute to the clinical signs and symptoms of sickle cell disease?

Damage to the endothelium (lining of the blood vessels) occurs in sickle cell disease. The red cells containing haemoglobin S have an increased adhesiveness (stickiness) and this can cause blockage to normal blood flow in these vessels.

KEY POINT

Decreased blood flow contributes significantly to the hypoxic organ damage. Emerging data indicate a role for disturbance of nitric oxide (NO) homeostasis in the pathogenesis of complications of sickle cell anaemia. Nitric oxide binds soluble guanylate cyclase which converts guanosine triphosphate (GTP) to cyclic guanosine monophosphate (cGMP), relaxing vascular smooth muscle and causing vasodilatation. Haemolysis of sickle erythrocytes releases free haemoglobin into the intravascular plasma compartment. This free haemoglobin in turn scavenges NO, altering the normal balance of vasomotor tone in the direction of vasoconstriction.

Complications of sickle cell disease including pulmonary hypertension, priapism, leg ulceration and stroke can all be linked to the intensity of haemolysis, which in turn correlates with NO consumption. It follows that agents that restore NO bioavailability or responsiveness may have the potential to reduce the incidence and severity of these complications. Drugs that modulate haemolysis and NO activity in sickle cell disease are now being evaluated in clinical trials.

What other clinical problems occur in patients with sickle cell disease?

Many clinical problems occur as a direct result of the abnormal haemoglobin in the red cells (Table 24; Fig. 53).

What else can be done to prevent these infectious complications?

Pneumococal vaccination and antibiotic prophylaxis (penicillin). This will reduce the risk of lethal infection. In young patients, stem cell transplantation is optional.

Recently, it has been shown that hydroxycarbamide, an inhibitor of ribonucleotide reductase, can significantly increase the level of fetal haemoglobin (Hb F) in patients with sickle cell disease. This will reduce the number of painful crises.

Table 24 Main clinical problems in individuals with sickle cell disease.

Stroke in young patients	Caused by occlusion of the blood vessels
Dactylitis in young children	Caused by bone marrow necrosis in the hands and the feet.
	The blood supply to the marrow is reduced because of the sickle cells
Severe infection	Splenic infarction because of the reduced blood supply caused by the sickle cells. Reduced splenic function increases the risk of infection with encapsulated bacteria, e.g. *Streptococcus pneumoniae*
Pregnancy	Pre-eclampsia because of sickle cells in the placental blood supply. This may also cause abortion
Avascular necrosis of the head of the femur	The blood supply is impaired because of the 'sickling' of the red cells
Priapism	Painful erections in males caused by 'sickling' and stagnation of blood in the penis
Folate deficiency	Chronic haemolysis may lead to a further fall in Hb.
	Patients should take folate supplements indefinitely
Gall stones	Chronic haemolysis increases the bilirubin turnover and may cause 'pigment' stones

---

KEY POINT

Frequent blood transfusion in children will reduce the risk of stroke.

Can you now construct an algorithm to investigate an individual of African descent with anaemia and a history of blood transfusion?

Yes.

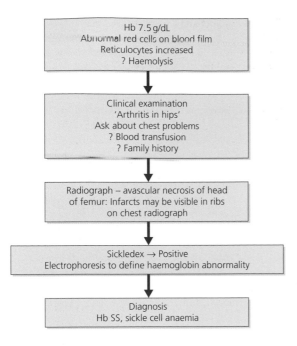

Hb 7.5 g/dL
Abnormal red cells on blood film
Reticulocytes increased
? Haemolysis

↓

Clinical examination
'Arthritis in hips'
Ask about chest problems
? Blood transfusion
? Family history

↓

Radiograph – avascular necrosis of head
of femur: Infarcts may be visible in ribs
on chest radiograph

↓

Sickledex → Positive
Electrophoresis to define haemoglobin abnormality

↓

Diagnosis
Hb SS, sickle cell anaemia

Outcome. Ola made a slow recovery. His temperature returned to normal and his breathing and chest radiograph gradually improved and the need for narcotic analgesia decreased. He was discharged from hospital 4 weeks later and was asked to attend the haematology clinic. He was given hydroxycarbamide in an attempt to reduce the number of painful crises and to reduce the need for blood transfusion.

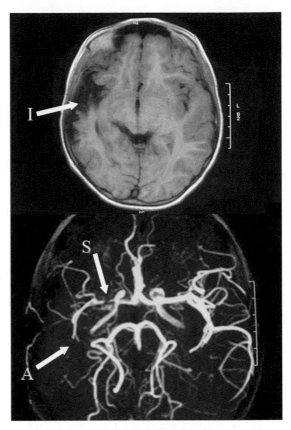

Figure 53 Brain infarct in a patient with Hb SS and a stroke. About 25% of patients with sickle cell disease develop cerebrovascular complications and about 80 of these are under 15 years of age. The magnetic resonance imaging (MRI) scan of the brain shows an area of infarction (I) secondary to vessel occlusion, stenosis (S) and absence (A).

CASE REVIEW

This young African man is acutely ill and requires immediate hospitalization and emergency treatment for respiratory insufficiency. Blood counts reveal severe anaemia and he gives a history of a diagnosis of Hb SS disease. This is confirmed by examination of a blood film and later by Hb electrophoresis.

The 'acute chest syndrome' seen in patients with Hb SS disease may be fatal and requires immediate treatment.

Antibiotic treatment is essential as many patients with Hb SS may have functional hyposplenism secondary to repeated splenic infarction. Hyposplenism may be obvious from the blood film with nucleated red cells, acanthocytes, target cells and Howell–Jolly bodies (nuclear fragments in

erythrocytes). Restoration of oxygen is paramount and this must be accompanied by correction of the anaemia to reduce the Hb SS to <30%. This can be achieved by blood transfusion but may require exchange transfusion.

Pain management is very important but care must be taken in the acute situation not to depress respiration with narcotic analgesics.

The patient should be encouraged to enrol with a hospital or primary care programme. Correct use of analgesia, early treatment of chest disease and adequate vaccination are important.

The use of the chemotherapeutic agent hydroxy-carbamide should be discussed with the patient.

KEY POINTS

- Hb SS disease results from a single crucial amino acid substitution in the globin chain
- Because of the altered solubility of Hb S, especially under conditions of reduced oxygen tension, the abnormal Hb will form precipitates within the erythrocytes
- This will result in decreased deformability and blood flow as well as increased blood viscosity causing ischaemic damage
- The myriad of possible clinical problems is outlined in Table 24
- More recently, the importance of nitric oxide has been recognized. Scavenging of this molecule by free Hb during a haemolytic episode contributes to vascular contraction making a 'bad' situation worse by further decreasing blood flow and increasing the possibility of ischaemia
- Active management of Hb SS disease in childhood by frequent blood transfusions and possibly the use of hydroxycarbamide may decrease the risk of stroke
- In spite of excellent medical facilities many patients with Hb SS disease die prematurely

Further reading

Hoffman R, Benze EJ Jr, Shattil SJ, Furie B, Cohen HJ, Silberstein LE, et al. eds. *Haematology: Basic Principles and Practice*, 4th edn. Churchill Livingstone, 2005: 605–644.

Miller ST, Sleeper LA, Pegelow CH, Enos LE, Wang WC, Weiner SJ, et al. Prediction of adverse outcomes in children with sickle cell disease. *New England Journal of Medicine* 2000; **342**: 83–89.

NHLBI. Sickle cell anemia. www.nhlbi.nih.gov/health/prof/blood/sickle/index.htm Accessed in 2006.

Rees DC, Olujohungbe AD, Parker NE, Stephens AD, Telfer P, Wright, British Committee for Standards in Haematology General Haematology Task Force by the Sickle Cell Working Party. Guidelines for the management of the acute painful crisis in sickle cell disease. *British Journal of Haematology* 2003; **120**: 744–752.

Rogers G, Telen MJ, Ataga KI, Ballas SK. Sickle cell anemia. Asheducationbook.hematologylibrary.org/cgi/content/full2007.

Wild BJ & Bain BJ. Investigation of abnormal haemoglobins and thalassaemia. In: Lewis SM, Bain BJ & Bates I, eds. *Dacie and Lewis: Practical Haematology*, 10th edn. Churchill Livingstone, 2006: 271–310.

A 19-year-old woman with thalassaemia

Luisa Corelli, a 19-year-old girl, has just moved to your locality from her native Sardinia. Luisa says she has a history of thalassaemia and needs follow-up care.

What steps should be taken to support the diagnosis?

A history and physical examination. Obtain full blood count (Table 25), blood film (Fig. 54) from the hospital in which the diagnosis was originally made and liver blood tests (Table 26).

Luisa says she commenced a chronic transfusion programme when she was aged 6. She requires red cell transfusion every 6–8 weeks. She has hypothyroidism and takes thyroxine replacement. She has been told recently that her blood glucose is slightly elevated. She is also taking an angiotensin converting enzyme (ACE) inhibitor for mild cardiac failure.

On examination Luisa was small in stature and her skin had a bronze colour. She had prominent frontal and parietal skull bones. The facial maxillae were enlarged. Her spleen was enlarged and palpable 2 cm below her left costal margin.

The differential white cell count was normal. The blood film (Fig. 54) showed hypochromic microcytic red cells, red cell fragments, nucleated red cells and polychromasia. Figure 55 shows the formation of blood cells in organs other than the marrow (liver, spleen and lymph nodes).

How can the physical examination and the blood results be explained?

The bronze colour could be explained by iron deposition in the skin but the blood film suggests a reduction in the amount of haemoglobin in each red cell and evidence of haemolysis (polychromasia, nucleated red cells and an elevated reticulocyte count). The large spleen is caused by a combination of haemolysis and extramedullary haemopoiesis.

What condition could thalassaemia be confused with on the basis of the red cell indices?

Iron deficiency because it also presents with a low haemoglobin and decreased MCH and MCV but will not have the other red cell changes and will have a low serum ferritin whereas thalassaemia will have a normal or high serum ferritin. Examination of the blood film (Fig. 54) and serum ferritin estimation should distinguish the two conditions.

What does the term 'thalassaemia' mean?

Thalassaemia is a quantitative disorder of globin chain synthesis. There are two main types, α and β thalassaemia, depending on which pair of globin chains is synthesized ineffectively. Normally, globin chain synthesis is balanced and haemoglobin A, the predominant form of Hb, consists of two A and two B chains. Each newly synthesized chain will pair appropriately to form haemoglobin, which is soluble within the red cell. In the homozygous thalassaemic state unbalanced α or β globin chain synthesis causes accumulation of insoluble unpaired chains which are toxic to the red cell precursors and mature red cells inducing both ineffective erythropoiesis and a haemolytic anaemia. The β thalassaemias result from over 150 different mutations of the β globin genes, which decrease the production of β globin chains, either completely or partially. They are inherited as autosomal recessive genes in similar fashion to qualitative disorders of haemoglobin synthesis, e.g. Hb SS (Case 7).

Haematology: Clinical Cases Uncovered. By S. McCann, R. Foà, O. Smith and E. Conneally. Published 2009 by Blackwell Publishing, ISBN: 978-1-4051-8322-2

Table 25 Results of the full blood count at the time of diagnosis.

	Patient's results	Normal range
Hb	5.2 g/dL	11.5–16.4 g/dL
MCV	59 fL	83–98 fL (μm^3)
WBC	4.2×10^9/L	$3.5–11.0 \times 10^9$/L (10^3/μL)
Platelets	389×10^9/L	$140–450 \times 10^9$/L (10^3/μL)
Reticulocyte count	480×10^9/L	$50–100 \times 10^9$/L (0.5–1.5%)

Hb, haemoglobin; MCV, mean corpuscular volume; WBC, white blood cell count.

Table 26 Results of liver blood tests.

	Patient's results	Normal range
AST (SGOT)	47 IU/L	7–40 IU/L
Alkaline phosphatase	130 IU/L	40–120 IU/L
GGT	62 IU/L	10–55 IU/L
Random blood glucose	13.0 mmol/L	<11.1 mmol/L (<200 mg/mL)

AST(SGOT), aspartamine amino transferase; GGT, gamma glutamyl amino transferase.

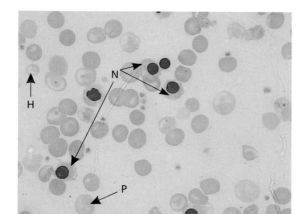

Figure 54 A blood film showing hypochromic (H), microcytic nucleated (N) red cells and polychromasia (P).

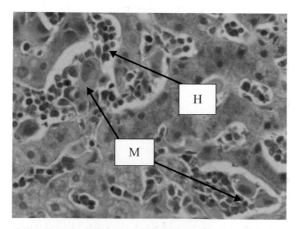

Figure 55 Extramedullary haemopoiesis: megakaryocytes (M); islands of haemopoiesis (H).

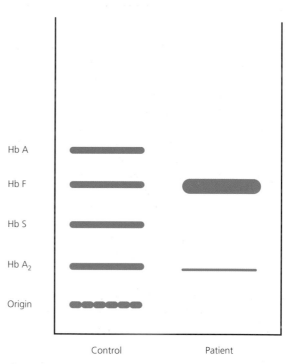

Figure 56 Haemoglobin electrophoresis showing the presence of Hb A_2, Hb F and absence of Hb A.

How was the diagnosis made originally?

Using haemoglobin electrophoresis to identify variant haemoglobins. This technique exposes proteins to a charge gradient and they are separated from each other by their size and charge (Fig. 56).

l *Bands of Hb A_2 and Hb F only were seen.*

Table 27 Different types of haemoglobin (Hb) during development.

Hb	Globin chains	Period when normally present
A	$\alpha_2\beta_2$	Major Hb in adult life
A$_2$	$\alpha_2\delta_2$	Minor Hb in adult life
F	$\alpha_2\gamma_2$	Minor Hb in adult life, major Hb in fetal life with declining % during neonatal period
Gower 1/2	$\zeta_2\varepsilon_2/\zeta_2\alpha_2$	Significant Hb during early intrauterine life
Portland 1/2	$\zeta_2\gamma_2/\zeta_2\beta_2$	Significant Hb during early intrauterine life

Table 28 Result of the serum ferritin.

	Patient's results	Normal range
Ferritin	3800 µg/L	20–300 µg/L (ng/mL)

What different haemoglobins are found in humans?

Each type of haemoglobin is composed of two different pairs of polypeptide chains (Table 27). The structure of haemoglobin changes during development. By 12 weeks' gestation, embryonic haemoglobin is replaced by fetal haemoglobin, which is slowly replaced after birth by the adult haemoglobins Hb A and Hb A$_2$. In adults, 96–98% of haemoglobin is haemoglobin A, which has two α chains and two β chains. Hb A has the structure of $\alpha_2\beta_2$ (two α chains and two β chains). The globin chains enfold a haem moiety consisting of a porphyrin ring complexed with a single iron atom. Each haem moiety can bind a single molecule of oxygen.

In view of the original blood and electrophoresis results what type of thalassemia did Luisa have?

Luisa has thalassaemia major because of the transfusion-dependent anaemia, splenomegaly and absence of Hb A on electrophoresis (β chains are necessary for the synthesis of Hb A).

What type of symptoms and haematological abnormalities exist in patients with β thalassaemia?

Heterozygotes for β thalassaemia (thalassaemia trait) are usually completely asymptomatic except in times of haemopoietic stress, e.g. during pregnancy. The blood count characteristically shows a normal or slightly reduced Hb, a reduction in the MCH and MCV and an elevated RBC count. The diagnosis depends upon the detection of an increased Hb A$_2$%. Homozygotes develop anaemia in the first year of life. The excess α chains precipitate in the red cell precursors leading to premature destruction. The bone marrow compensates by increasing the number of reticulocytes. This bone marrow expansion leads to changes in the skull and long bones.

Why might Luisa have hypothyroidism and elevated blood glucose?

Iron deposition in the endocrine organs.

How would this be confirmed?

Serum ferritin (Table 28).

Why might she be at risk of iron deposition in her organs and what other organs might be involved?

The major complication of thalassaemia is iron overload.

The excess iron becomes deposited in the tissues particularly the heart, liver and pancreas which if untreated can lead to cardiomyopathy, liver disease or diabetes mellitus. The human body has no effective way of removing excess iron other than bleeding.

> **KEY POINT**
>
> Each unit of red cells (250 mL) contains approximately 125 mg iron.

What other abnormalities or deficiencies could contribute to her anaemia?

Folate deficiency because of the chronic haemolysis.

All patients with significant degrees of thalassaemia should receive folate acid supplements on a daily basis indefinitely.

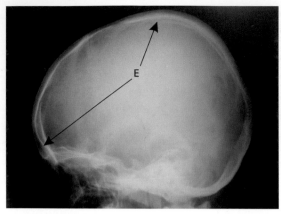

Figure 57 Skull radiograph showing expansion of the cranial bone marrow cavity caused by ineffective haematopoiesis (E). It is also called 'hair on end' appearance.

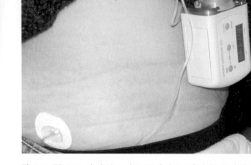

Figure 58 Iron chelation therapy being administered via an infusion pump.

How can the abnormal facial and skull appearance be explained?

Expansion of the marrow cavity in the skull and facial bones to compensate for the severe anaemia (Fig. 57).

What other complications of blood transfusions can you anticipate?

Transfusion transmitted viral infections are a major problem for thalassaemia patients who commenced their transfusion programme before blood donations were routinely tested for the viruses that cause hepatitis and AIDS. Chronic viral hepatitis and hepatic siderosis can act synergistically to promote chronic liver disease.

Her hepatitis B serology was negative and she was hepatitis C virus antibody (anti-HCV) positive, meaning she had been exposed to HCV. A subsequent test showed she was HCV RNA positive, demonstrating ongoing replication of HCV. Her HIV serology was negative. She should be vaccinated against hepatitis B and referred to a hepatologist.

In view of the above, what abnormalities of the liver blood tests would you expect?

Many patients with hepatitis C are asymptomatic and their liver blood tests are relatively normal. Chronic hepatitis occurs in about 50–70% of those infected with hepatitis C. Among asymptomatic people with anti-HCV, 33–50% have evidence of inflammation on liver biopsy.

What are the principles of treatment?

Red cell transfusion to relieve anaemia, iron chelation and consideration of the possibility of allogeneic stem cell transplantation if a suitable donor is available.

How should iron overload be treated?

Phlebotomy is the most efficient and least toxic way of removing excess iron; however, it is not applicable in someone like Luisa who is anaemic. The most effective method of iron chelation is desferrioxamine, which binds iron and promotes its excretion in the urine. It has to be administered by continuous subcutaneous infusion for 8–12 hours/day (Fig. 58).

Luisa has been prescribed desferrioxamine, via subcutaneous infusion, 5 nights per week for 12 hours. She admits that over the last few years she has missed some of the doses as it interferes with her lifestyle.

> **KEY POINT**
>
> Because of difficulties with compliance and toxicity (retinal damage) associated with desferrioxamine, oral iron chelators are currently being evaluated. Two oral compounds are used (deferiprone and deferasirox), one causing increased excretion of iron in the urine and the other in the faeces. Agranulocytosis has been reported in 1% of users of the latter. Endocrine replacement therapy may be required.

Three months later Luisa attends the surgery acutely unwell. She has a 2-day history of right upper quadrant colicky abdominal pain and nausea. She has a tachycardia of 120 beats/minute. She has a temperature of 38.5°C and is acutely tender in the right upper quadrant with guarding and localized rebound tenderness.

What might explain these symptoms and signs?

Acute cholecystitis (inflammation of the gallbladder).

Why should a patient of her age develop cholecystitis?

Patients with chronic haemolytic anaemia (as part of her thalassaemia syndrome) are more likely to have pigment gallstones. Acute inflammation of the gallbladder usually follows obstruction of the cystic duct by a stone.

The presence of increased amounts of insoluble bilirubin in bile results in the precipitation of the bilirubin which aggregates and forms pigment stones.

Can you now construct an algorithm for a patient with severe microcytic hypochromic anaemia?

Yes.

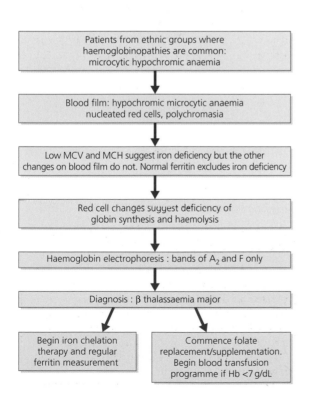

Outcome. Luisa was admitted to hospital where the diagnosis of acute cholecystitis was confirmed. An abdominal ultrasound confirmed the presence of stones. She was treated with intravenous antibiotics for 3 days; however, she remained very ill. A laparotomy and cholecystectomy were performed. Postoperatively she developed acute heart failure, which was felt to be secondary to a cardiomyopathy from her iron overload. She was treated with diuretics but unfortunately continued to deteriorate. She died in the intensive care unit 48 hours after surgery.

CASE REVIEW

A young girl presents with a known history of thalassaemia. She has the typical physical features of chronic ineffective erythropoiesis and extramedullary haemopoiesis. From the history it appears that the girl may not have adequate iron chelation therapy therefore clinical management must assess the degree of anaemia, the requirement for red cell transfusion and effective iron chelation. Complications of ineffective erythropoiesis and premature red cell destruction must be sought. Transmission of infectious agents from blood transfusion must be investigated.

The findings of severe anaemia requiring blood transfusion and the investigations confirm a diagnosis of β thalassaemia. She has evidence of hepatitis C, most probably from blood transfusion, which she received before adequate testing was mandatory.

She has clinical evidence of iron overload with diabetes, cardiac failure and hypothyroidism. Treatment is aimed at maintaining an adequate haemoglobin, making sure she is adequately chelated to prevent and possibly reverse some of the toxicity of iron. Treatment of the complications, in this case gallstones, is important.

Because of inadequate iron chelation she has significant iron deposition in her heart and dies from this coupled with the stress of infection and anaesthesia. The development of new oral iron chelators should increase compliance by patients.

Stem cell transplantation has been demonstrated to be very effective with a low mortality. This form of therapy is expensive, complicated and requires matched sibling donors.

KEY POINTS

- The clinical presentation of this condition varies widely depending on the quantitative deficiency in globin chain synthesis. The gene deletion has clinical manifestations which vary from a slightly reduced haemoglobin (α thalassaemia with a single gene deletion) to death *in utero* from hydrops fetalis (absence of four α chain genes)
- Quantitative haemoglobinopathies can exist in combination with qualitative defects (e.g. Hb SA, Hb CA) and the clinical effects will be modified accordingly
- Antenatal diagnosis is offered in some countries and therapeutic abortion may be a consideration in countries where it is legal
- The disease is common worldwide but in many countries health services are inadequate to provide accurate diagnosis and treatment to all patients. Inadequate screening of blood to prevent viral transmission through transfusion may also be a problem for poorly developed health services
- The major cause of morbidity and mortality is the result of iron overload and its sequelae

Further reading

Beris P, Brissot P, Cappellini M. Iron metabolism and related disorders. www.ironcurriculum.esh.org/ Accessed in 2008.

Borgna-Pignatti C & Galannello R. The thalassaemias and related disorders: quantitative disorders of haemoglobin synthesis. In: *Wintrobe's Clinical Haematology*, 11th edn, Vol. 1. Lippincott, Williams and Wilkins, 2004.

Hoffbrand AV, Pettit JE & Moss PAH. *Essential Haematology*, 5th edn. Blackwell Science, Oxford, 2006.

Olivieri NF. The β-thalassemias. *New England Journal of Medicine* 1999; **341**: 99–109.

Weatherall DJ & Clegg JB. *The Thalassaemia Syndromes*, 4th edn. Blackwell Science, Oxford, 2001.

Wild BJ & Bain BJ. Investigation of abnormal haemoglobins and thalassaemia. In: Lewis SM, Bain BJ & Bates I, eds. *Dacie and Lewis: Practical Haematology*, 10th edn. Churchill Livingstone, 2006: 271–310.

Case 9 · A 17-year-old boy with a sore throat and bleeding gums

A mother brought her 17-year-old boy, Anatole, to the family doctor because he had a sore throat, bleeding from his gums and a rash on his ankles. He had vomited on three occasions the evening before and had developed two red eyes. He was a schoolboy and denied cigarette smoking, alcohol intake or using recreational drugs. Anatole had been perfectly well until 3 weeks before.

The family doctor noted a red appearance in Anatole's throat, bilateral subconjunctival haemorrhages and some petechiae on his legs. The family doctor was unable to palpate any lymph nodes or enlargement of the liver or spleen. His temperature was elevated at 38°C. He looked pale.

What is your differential diagnosis?

A sore throat suggests infection, which is commonly caused by a viral infection and less commonly by infection with streptococcus. The presence of white exudates on the tonsils suggests but is not diagnostic of bacterial infection. Pallor suggests anaemia, which you would not expect in an otherwise healthy young boy. The presence of subconjunctival bleeding and petechiae would suggest a low platelet count. Severe vomiting can cause subconjunctival bleeding in normal individuals but its presence following three episodes of vomiting together with purpura should alert you to something more serious.

The symptoms and signs suggest that the bone marrow (the factory that produces blood) may not be functioning properly and the production of red cells and platelets is deficient. The findings could also be explained by premature destruction of red cells and platelets.

A serious illness such as leukaemia or aplastic anaemia should be suspected.

Haematology: Clinical Cases Uncovered. By S. McCann, R. Foà, O. Smith and E. Conneally. Published 2009 by Blackwell Publishing, ISBN: 978-1-4051-8322-2

What should be done next?

Arrange for Anatole to be seen immediately by a haematologist or otherwise attend the accident and emergency department at the nearest hospital.

What therapeutic approach should be taken to treat his fever?

In adults it is rarely necessary to treat a fever. However, in young children high fevers can cause febrile convulsions and should be treated.

Which antipyretic would you use if required?

Paracetamol. Aspirin should not be given to a patient with a low platelet count.

> **KEY POINT**
>
> Aspirin interferes with platelet function (it does not alter platelet numbers) through its inhibition of cyclo-oxygenase and can initiate bleeding (especially if the platelet count is low).

Why should intramuscular injections be avoided?

They can cause bleeding into the muscle (haematoma) in the presence of a low platelet count and should not be used until the platelet count had been measured. In the case of a suspected low platelet count or abnormal platelet function, all medications should be given by mouth or intravenously.

Anatole arrived at the accident and emergency department of the hospital 1 hour later with a letter from the family doctor.

What should the doctor on duty do?

Take a detailed medical history asking about any recent travel, medications and use of recreational drugs or possible exposure to infection with viruses including HIV. A history of jaundice should be specifically enquired about.

As stated to the family doctor there were no medications. Anatole denied foreign travel and use of recreational drugs or exposure to possible HIV infection.

Why should his mother be excluded for the interview?

The presence of the patient's mother might inhibit the patient from admitting to the use of recreational drugs or exposure to HIV infection (Part 1b).

Following the history the doctor examined Anatole and confirmed the findings of the family doctor without additional abnormalities (Figs 59 and 60).

What should the doctor do next?

A blood count (Table 29), coagulation screen and a liver, renal and bone profile, urinalysis, blood pressure and chest radiograph.

I *There was a trace of haemolysed blood in the urine.*

How can these blood findings be interpreted?

A decrease in the haemoglobin, white cell and platelet count is known as pancytopenia.

The fact that the red cells are larger than normal (elevated MCV) suggests a defect in the maturation of the red cells in the bone marrow or an increase in the number of young circulating red cells known as reticulocytes. However, a low reticulocyte count suggests a difficulty in manufacturing red cells. The reduced neutrophil and platelet count suggests that the production problem might also be affecting these cells.

In view of the elevated MCV (macrocytosis), blood should be sent for an estimation of serum vitamin B_{12} and red cell folate.

Table 29 Results of the blood tests.

	Patient's results	Normal range (male)
Hb	8.9 g/dL	13.5–18.0 g/dL
Red cell count	3.0×10^{12}/L	4.60–5.70×10^{12}/L (10^6/μL)
MCV	103 fL	83–99 fL (μm³)
WBC	2.2×10^9/L	4.0–11.0×10^9/L (10^3/μL)
Platelets	18×10^9/L	140–450×10^9/L (10^3/μL)
Neutrophils	0.2×10^9/L	2.0–7.5×10^9/L (10^3/μL)
Lymphocytes	2.3×10^9/L	1.5–3.5×10^9/L (10^3/μL)
Reticulocytes	24×10^9/L	50–100×10^9/L (0.5–1.5%)

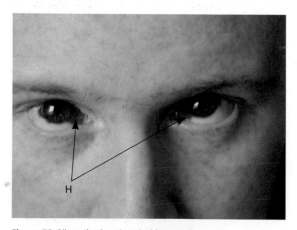

Figure 59 Bilateral subconjunctival haemorrhages (H).

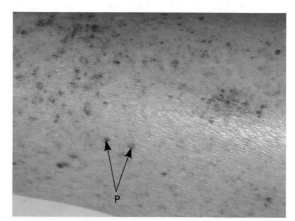

Figure 60 Petechial rash on the leg.

How does this blood picture help you to interpret the physical findings in the patient?

The low platelet count explains the rash on Anatole's legs (purpura) and the subconjunctival bleeding following a bout of vomiting.

> **KEY POINT**
>
> Bleeding may occur after minor trauma if the platelet count is below 50×10^9/L. Bleeding may occur spontaneously if the platelet count goes below 10×10^9/L.

The raised intracranial pressure (as a result of the vomiting) precipitated the boy's subconjunctival bleeding. Subconjunctival bleeding is of no danger to the patient's vision. It alerts us to the presence of a low platelet count and unless prompt corrective action is taken quickly, there is a risk of intracranial bleeding. The retina should be examined immediately for fresh haemorrhages. Retinal haemorrhages can interfere with vision especially if they occur in the area of the macula. It is important to measure the blood pressure when the platelet count is low. The presence of an elevated systolic blood pressure significantly increases the risk of serious retinal or intracranial bleeding and should be treated as an emergency. In this case the blood pressure was within normal limits. The rash on the legs is a result of bleeding into the skin, known as purpura, which is caused by the low platelet count. Purpura can be confluent, in which case it is called a bruise or ecchymosis, or it can be punctate and appear as small red dots like pinpoints. These dots are known as petechiae. The reason that this type of bleeding occurs predominantly in the legs is simply due to increased hydrostatic pressure in the small blood vessels of the skin when walking.

The doctor examined Anatole's retina and there were no haemorrhages. The trace of blood in his urine can occur with a low platelet count and was not considered to indicate renal pathology. The coagulation, biochemical screens and chest radiograph were normal.

Why was the coagulation screen normal?

The coagulation screen is not influenced by the platelet count.

> **KEY POINT**
>
> The role of the patient's platelet count is overridden by the addition of a substitute for the platelet phospholipid in the prothrombin time (PT) and the activated partial thromboplastin time (APTT).

What should the doctor do next?

Admit the patient to hospital immediately and arrange a bone marrow aspirate and biopsy.

How should the bone marrow aspirate and biopsy be approached to prevent bleeding?

There is no need to give platelets prior to the aspiration and biopsy of marrow from the posterior iliac crest. Firm digital pressure should be applied for 5 minutes or until the bleeding stops. A firm pressure dressing should then be applied and inspected 30 minutes later for bleeding (Figs 61 and 62).

Pressure dressings should be small and tightly applied. Large dressings will only obscure bleeding and rarely exert adequate pressure.

The bone marrow aspirate was reported as 'hypoplastic', with a few marrow cells present but no abnormal cells were seen. No megaloblastic features were present to suggest a deficiency of vitamin B_{12} or folic acid. The marrow biopsy also revealed severe hypoplasia and again no abnormal cells were seen.

The vitamin B_{12} and folate levels were normal.

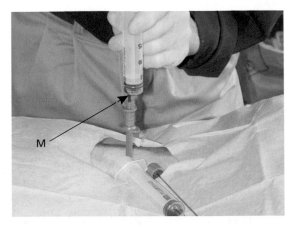

Figure 61 Bone marrow (M) being aspirated from the posterior iliac crest.

PART 2: CASES

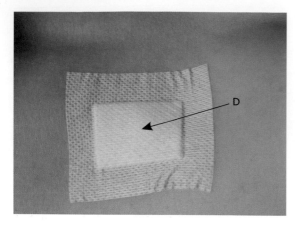

Figure 62 A pressure dressing (D) applied to the aspirate site.

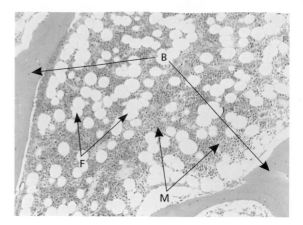

Figure 63 Normal marrow biopsy. Marrow cells (M) are seen between the fat spaces (F). Bony trebeculae are pink (B).

Vitamin B_{12} deficiency would be extremely rare in a patient of this age. Folate deficiency could be present secondary to coeliac disease. In folate or vitamin B_{12} deficiency causing a pancytopenia, the biochemical screen would be abnormal with elevated levels of bilirubin and lactic dehydrogenase indicating ineffective erythropoiesis (premature destruction of haemopoietic cells in the marrow) and the red cell and white cell precursors would show megaloblastic change (Case 3).

The marrow aspirate and biopsy complement each other. The aspirate allows us to examine individual cells in detail and the biopsy allows us to assess the marrow architecture. The biopsy is especially useful in assessing the cellularity of the marrow and the presence of non-haemopoietic cells such as metastatic cancer (Figs 63 and 64).

Now what is your differential diagnosis?

Because the marrow biopsy reveals a severe reduction in the number of marrow cells present and there is no evidence of abnormal cells, the diagnosis is aplastic anaemia. Occasionally, acute leukaemia may present with an 'aplastic phase' and the correct diagnosis may only become obvious after some months.

Aplastic anaemia is a rare condition in which the marrow elements are severely reduced in the absence of abnormal cells. Although drugs and viral infections rarely precede the onset of aplastic anaemia, the aetiology is unknown in the majority of cases (Table 30).

There is laboratory and clinical evidence to suggest that in most cases the pathogenesis of aplastic anaemia is autoimmune.

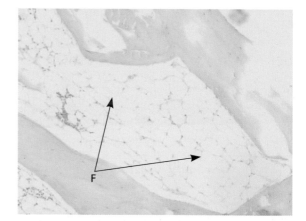

Figure 64 Marrow biopsy from a patient with severe aplastic anaemia. Most of the normal marrow is replaced by fat spaces (F).

In clinical practice you rarely find any cause for aplastic anaemia. A virus is rarely incriminated as a causal agent even if liver blood tests suggest a recent viral infection.

KEY POINT

The spleen is not enlarged in patients with aplastic anaemia. If the spleen is enlarged another explanation for the pancytopenia should be sought.

Table 30 Drugs and viruses linked to aplastic anaemia.

Drugs linked to aplastic anaemia	Viruses linked to aplastic anaemia
Chloramphenicol	Epstein–Barr virus
Co-trimoxazole	Hepatitis B virus
Chloroquin	HIV virus
Anti inflammatories	
Gold salts	
Penicillamine	
Carbimazole	
Phenothiazines	
Carbamazepine	
Phenytoin	

What are the principles of treatment?

Patients rarely recover and in the severe forms of the disease the majority of patients will die from infection or bleeding within a few months unless the underlying defect is corrected. The most effective treatment for severe aplastic anaemia is sibling (brother or sister) stem cell transplantation.

KEY POINT

The patient receives 'conditioning' with large doses of cyclophosphamide followed by an intravenous infusion of stem cells from the donor's bone marrow. The donor stem cells differentiate and produce blood cells in about 2–3 weeks. The major cause of morbidity and mortality is graft versus host disease (GvHD).

What alternative treatment is available if a family donor is not found?

Treatment with powerful immunosuppressive agents (antithymocyte globulin and cyclosporine without giving stem cells) is frequently effective (up to 70%).

Results of stem cell transplantation with carefully matched unrelated donors and powerful immunosuppression of the recipient have improved and may become

the treatment of choice in young patients with severe aplastic anaemia if a fully matched sibling donor is not available.

Which inherited conditions manifest as aplastic anaemia?

The most common of these rare conditions is Fanconi's anaemia. This disorder is associated with two genetic abnormalities on chromosome 9 and 16, which leads to defective DNA repair. Clinically, there are often many abnormalities including short stature, pigmentation, skeletal and renal abnormalities and aplastic anaemia. Those affected have an increased risk of developing acute myeloid leukaemia and solid tumours.

Can you construct an algorithm to investigate a patient with pancytopenia?

Yes.

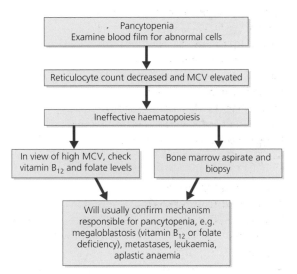

Outcome. The patient had a human leucocyte antigen (HLA) compatible sister and he received a bone marrow transplant within 1 month of his diagnosis. His transplant was uncomplicated and he is now a final year medical student.

Bone marrow transplantation successfully cures >80% of young adults with aplastic anaemia if a compatible family donor is available.

CASE REVIEW

A 17-year-old boy presents with evidence of bone marrow failure (anaemia, infection and bleeding). He is clearly ill and needs rapid expert investigation and management. Urgent transfer to a haematology department should be undertaken as management is complicated. Because of the combination of anaemia, bleeding and infection he probably has a serious underlying blood disease such as leukaemia or aplastic anaemia.

Infection in people with very low neutrophil counts commonly develops into septicaemia and requires treatment with high doses of intravenous antibiotics even

before a pathogen is isolated. Severe anaemia and bleeding should be treated with red cell and platelet transfusions. If stem cell transplantation is contemplated, transfusions should be kept to a minimum to avoid sensitization and possible graft rejection.

The severity of the bleeding needs expert assessment and management to avoid intracranial haemorrhage. Examination of the bone marrow is critical and provides the diagnosis. Stem cell transplantation is the treatment of choice for severe aplastic anaemia and the patient should be referred to a transplant centre for assessment.

KEY POINTS

- Aplastic anaemia is a rare disease. It can be rapidly fatal unless managed expertly
- Bleeding into the skin (purpura) suggests a low platelet count, abnormal platelet function or inflammation of blood vessels (vasculitis). This is often accompanied by bleeding into mucosal surfaces (e.g. lining of gastrointestinal tract or uterus)
- In contrast, bleeding into joints or muscles usually indicates a coagulopathy
- Inhibition of platelet function by aspirin is *irreversible* and therefore will not be corrected until all affected platelets have died
- Platelet lifespan is 5–7 days
- Paroxysmal nocturnal haemoglobinuria (PNH) is a rare acquired stem cell disorder where the *PIG A* gene is

defective. This results in the lack of binding of a number of factors, which inhibit the effect of complement on the red cell. Consequently, when complement is activated, red cells are lysed in the circulation. Some patients present with signs and symptoms of bone marrow failure similar to aplastic anaemia
- When using stem cell transplantation for patients with severe aplastic anaemia, donor stem cells from bone marrow rather than peripheral blood should be used as the risk of GvHD is less
- Patients should be transferred to a haematology department as quickly as possible after a diagnosis as rapid treatment increases the chance of a successful outcome

Further reading

Hoffbrand AV, Moss PAH & Pettit JE. *Essential Haematology*, 5th edn. Blackwell Science, Oxford, 2006: 241–248.

Marsh JCW, Ball SE, Darbyshire P, *et al*. Guidelines for the diagnosis and management of acquired aplastic anaemia. *British Journal of Haematology* 2003; **123**: 782–801.

Schrezenmeier H & Bacigalupo A, eds. *Aplastic Anaemia: Pathophysiology and Treatment*. Cambridge University Press, 1999.

Young NS & Beris P. Acquired aplastic anemias. *Seminars in Haematology* 2000; **37**: 1.

Young NS & Maciejewski JP. Aplastic anemia. In: Hoffman R, Benz EJ, Shattil SJ, Furie B, Cohen HJ, Silverstein LE, *et al*. eds. *Hematology: Basic Principles and Practice*, 4th edn. Churchill Livingstone, 2004: 381–417.

A 33-year-old football player who was dropped from the team

Nasir Khan, a 33-year-old pharmaceutical hospital specialist, was 'dropped' from the football team. He admitted to the coach that he had been feeling unusually tired for the last 6 months and had occasional episodes of sweating, especially at night. He went to his family doctor.

The only additional symptom that Nasir mentioned was occasional discomfort in his left upper abdomen. He did not smoke or consume alcohol. He had never been in hospital, was taking no medications and denied use of recreational drugs.

What might be causing his symptoms?

Fatigue could be caused by anaemia or depression, and 'sweating' could be a manifestation of infection.

How is sweating evaluated?

Ask: 'Did you have to change your bed clothes because of the night sweat?'

Anxiety, hyperthyroidism, infections (e.g. tuberculosis) and some haematological malignancies (e.g. non-Hodgkin's lymphoma, chronic myeloid leukaemia) can cause sweating. A travel history should be taken because infections (such as malaria), not commonly seen in Europe, can present in this way. A full physical examination should be undertaken.

What should be done next?

A full physical examination.

Nasir appeared healthy. There was no evidence of weight loss and the only abnormal finding was an enlarged spleen, palpable 4 cm below the left costal margin on quiet inspiration. There was no lymphadenopathy and his chest was clinically clear.

Haematology: Clinical Cases Uncovered. By S. McCann, R. Foà, O. Smith and E. Conneally. Published 2009 by Blackwell Publishing, ISBN: 978-1-4051-8322-2

Where is the spleen in a healthy individual?

The spleen lies between the 9th and 11th ribs posteriorly. It is not normally palpable. Occasionally in a very thin individual you may be able to palpate the tip of the spleen on deep inspiration.

In this case the spleen was easily palpable in quiet inspiration and therefore is significantly enlarged (Fig. 65).

What is your differential diagnosis?

A palpable spleen in an otherwise healthy looking young man suggests either a haematological disorder or an increase in blood flow through the spleen causing it to enlarge (e.g. portal hypertension). Haematological disorders include non-Hodgkin's lymphoma, Hodgkin's lymphoma, chronic myeloid leukaemia, autoimmune haemolytic anaemia, a congenital haemolytic anaemia and hairy cell leukaemia. Myelofibrosis causes splenic enlargement but would be very unusual in a patient of this age. In tropical areas, infections such as malaria and schistosomiasis may cause a large spleen. Chronic liver disease with portal hypertension will cause enlargement of the spleen but there are usually other signs and symptoms of liver disease present.

How reliable is physical examination in assessing spleen size?

It is reliable for an experienced examiner. However, in obese individuals it may be very difficult to feel a slightly enlarged spleen.

What investigation will define the size of the spleen?

Ultrasound examination of the abdomen is a reliable non-invasive inexpensive test (Fig. 66).

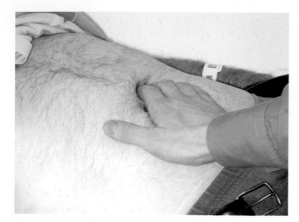

Figure 65 Palpation of a large spleen extending below the left lower ribs.

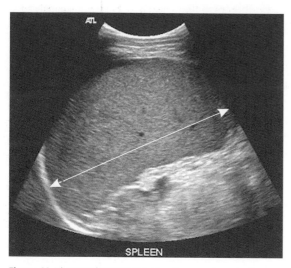

Figure 66 Ultrasound examination showing an enlarged spleen (the dark grey area outlined by the arrow) measuring 13.8 cm (normal: 11–12 cm).

What investigations might help to find the cause of the enlarged spleen?

A full blood count, blood film, reticulocyte count and a biochemical screen (Tables 31 and 32).

> There was a marked increase in the white cell count. White cell precursors including metamyelocytes, myelocytes and promyelocytes were present (Fig. 67).

Now what is the differential diagnosis?

The haemoglobin is normal and the white cell count is elevated. White cell precursors are present. These cells

Table 31 Results of the full blood and reticulocyte count.

	Patient's results	Normal range (male)
Hb	14.0 g/dL	13.5–18.0 g/dL
WBC	55.0×10^9/L	$4.0–11.0 \times 10^9$/L (10^3/µL)
Platelets	600×10^9/L	$140–450 \times 10^9$/L (10^3/µL)
Reticulocyte count	64.0×10^9/L	$50–100 \times 10^9$/L (0.5–1.5%)

Hb, haemoglobin; WBC, white blood cell count.

Table 32 Results of the lactic dehydrogenase (LDH) and urate (uric acid) tests.

	Patient's results	Normal range
LDH	850 IU/L	230–450 IU/L
Urate (uric acid)	600 µmol/L	150–470 µmol/L (3–8 mg/dL)

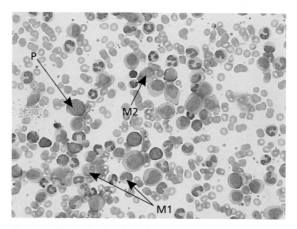

Figure 67 Blood film showing white cell precursors, metamyelocytes (M1), myelocytes (M2) and promyelocytes (P).

are normally found in the bone marrow and not in the peripheral blood. The platelet count is also elevated. This suggests that the bone marrow is overactive and releasing white cells and platelets prematurely into the circulation. The results of these tests therefore suggest a severe disturbance of the bone marrow rather than an infectious disease.

The most likely diagnosis is chronic myeloid leukaemia.

The blood findings are typical and there is no lymphadenopathy to suggest a lymphoma. There is no evidence of severe infection or liver disease.

What should be done next?

Nasir should be referred to a haematologist because he probably has a significant haematological disorder.

He received an appointment to see a haematologist 2 days later. Nasir was advised not to play football and to avoid strenuous exercise until he had been seen by the haematologist.

Why was this advice given?

It is possible to rupture an enlarged spleen following trauma. This could lead to life-threatening intra-abdominal bleeding.

Nasir was interviewed and examined by the haematologist who repeated the blood count and blood film and received the results of the biochemical screen and ultrasound examination.

How are the biochemical results explained?

The elevated lactic dehydrogenase (LDH) reflects cell death and is non-specific. It could be elevated following myocardial infarction, liver damage or premature death of blood cells. In this case it reflects death of white blood cells. Similarly, the elevated uric acid level in the plasma reflects increased cell turnover.

What should be done next?

A bone marrow examination was arranged because a serious haematological disorder was suspected.

From which site was the bone marrow aspirated?

The posterior iliac crest. It is the least painful site for the patient and almost completely without hazard. Care should be taken to make sure that adequate local analgesia is given and that there is no bleeding after the procedure.

What investigations would the haematologist request on the sample of bone marrow?

Slides for microscopic examination. A sample should be also sent to the genetics department for a karyotypic (cytogenetic) analysis and/or fluorescence *in situ* hybridization (FISH).

How does the bone marrow aspirate help to confirm the suspected diagnosis?

The slides revealed a very cellular specimen with increased numbers of white blood cell and platelet precursors (megakaryocytes) suggesting increased marrow activity or reduced cell death (apoptosis). There are no specific abnormalities in the bone marrow in most patients with chronic myeloid leukaemia (CML) at diagnosis other than an increase in cellularity.

What other marrow specimens should the doctor or nurse practitioner obtain?

A biopsy of the bone marrow (Figs 68 and 69), also from the posterior iliac crest, will yield complementary information.

How should the patient be managed?

The probable diagnosis should be explained to Nasir. If he had a partner he/she should be invited, with the patient's permission, to come back in a few days

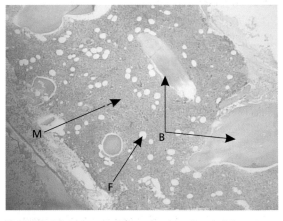

Figure 68 A bone marrow biopsy showing a hypercellular marrow (M). Bony trabeculae are shown in pink (B). Fat spaces are reduced (F).

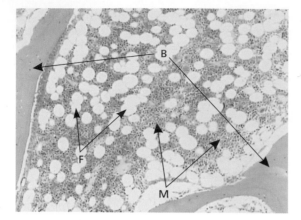

Figure 69 A normal bone marrow biopsy showing bone marrow cells (M), bony trabeculae (B) and fat spaces (F).

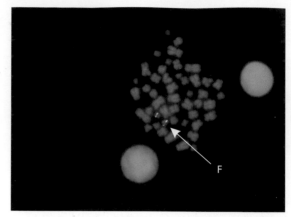

Figure 71 Fluorescence *in situ* hybridization (FISH) analysis of bone marrow cells showing the 9:22 translocation (F).

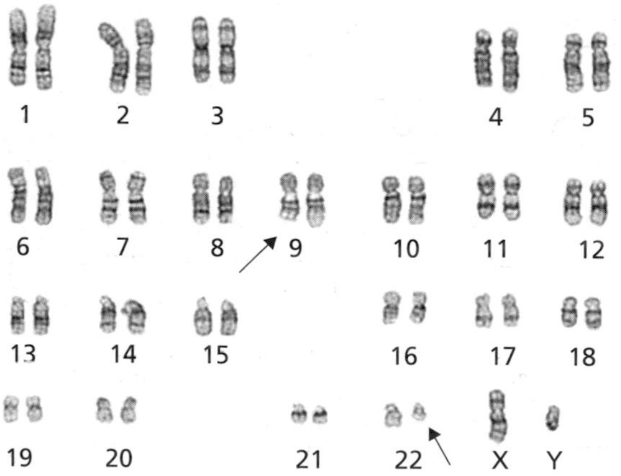

Figure 70 The abnormally small chromosome 22, the 'Philadelphia' chromosome.

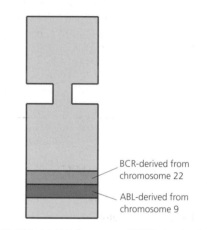

Figure 72 'Philadelphia' chromosome t(9:22), showing the two chromosomal fragments together on chromosome 22, results in the synthesis of a protein which causes the leukaemia cells to behave in a malignant way.

to discuss the result of the outstanding tests. The patient should be assured that there is no immediate danger, but be advised to remain off work and refrain from contact sports until the diagnosis is clarified.

What medications would the haematologist prescribe?

Nasir was advised to take allopurinol, a competitive inhibitor of xanthine oxidase. This drug will reduce the level of urate (uric acid) in the plasma and decrease the risk of gout and renal damage.

The patient and his partner were given the results 3 days later.

The cytogenetic analysis revealed a normal number of chromosomes but a small chromosome 22 (Fig. 70). This was because of a translocation of a portion of chromosome 9 to chromosome 22 and a reciprocal (reverse) transfer of a portion of chromosome from chromosome 22 to chromosome 9 (Fig. 71).

Why is this small chromosome 22 called the 'Philadelphia chromosome' and what is its significance?

Two scientists in Philadelphia first described the small abnormal chromosome 22 in patients with CML. This translocation was the first non-random reproducible chromosomal abnormality to be described in a human cancer. It is always present in the bone marrow cells of patients with CML. It is very significant in our understanding of the pathogenesis of CML. When portions of different chromosomes come together the production of an abnormal gene product (protein) occurs. In the case of CML the abnormal gene product influences cell division and programmed cell death (apoptosis). The fusion gene on chromosome 22 is called *BCR/ABL* (Fig. 72).

KEY POINT

The abnormal chromosome found in CML produces an oncoprotein which causes the malignant phenotype, i.e. makes the cells behave in a cancerous way. The cells have altered adherence in the bone marrow and are very resistant to apoptosis (programmed cell death). This knowledge has stimulated the development of drugs that specifically inhibit these abnormalities and induce apoptosis of the leukaemia cells resulting in a remission of the disease.

What should the haematologist tell the patient and his partner?

Reassure Nasir and his partner that there is no immediate danger and that all his symptoms will disappear following 3–4 weeks of treatment.

What is the long-term outlook for the patient?

Current therapy of first choice involves the drug imatinib mesylate, a tyrosine kinase inhibitor (TKI). This agent is taken by mouth and has a relatively low toxicity profile. It inhibits the ATP binding site on the *BCR/ABL* gene and thus interferes with phosphorylation of a number of intracellular signal transduction factors. The majority of patients have a response to this drug, which includes normalization of their blood counts, relief from symptoms and disappearance of the Philadelphia chromosome from the blood and bone marrow. In most patients the response is long-lived; however, there is a requirement for continued therapy. Therefore the requirement for stem cell transplantation has acutely diminished since 2000. Patients who are intolerant or resistant to imatinib may respond to so-called second

generation TKIs. These drugs are more potent, toxic and expensive.

Can you construct an algorithm for investigation of a patient with a high white cell count and a large spleen?

Yes.

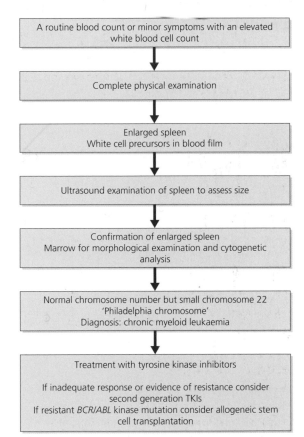

Outcome. Imatinib mesylate, a new agent capable of inducing apoptosis in the leukaemia cells, was prescribed. Nasir returned to work in a few days and was able to resume a normal life.

He is seen in the haematology clinic at monthly intervals. He remains well 4 years later. The Philadelphia chromosome can no longer be found in his blood or bone marrow and the molecular marker of his disease (BCR/ABL transcripts) are no longer identifiable. Nasir no longer plays football but his exercise capacity is normal.

CASE REVIEW

A young man presents with non-specific symptoms but because he had been dropped from the football team there was probably something significant going on. The most important finding was splenomegaly, which is never a normal finding.

Your differential diagnosis will be influenced by observing if the patient is ill, has evidence of liver disease and his/her ethnic background. Haemoglobinopathies such as thalassaemia and some infectious diseases are seen in certain populations and mass travel has exposed many people to infectious diseases.

The blood counts are indicative of the underlying diagnosis and bone marrow morphology does not add much additional information. The critical test is the genetic analysis. The translocation, t(9:22), is found in all patients with CML and a few patients with acute lymphoblastic leukaemia.

Having made a diagnosis of CML the treatment was, until recently, allogeneic stem cell transplantation. The development of an orally available drug that is specifically aimed at the chimaeric gene represents a major breakthrough. TKI treatment is now the approach in newly diagnosed patients, with stem cell transplantation reserved for a minority who do not respond or who are intolerant of TKIs.

KEY POINTS

- t(9:22) was the first non-random chromosomal translocation to be found in human malignancy
- The translocation is important because the oncoprotein produced causes the malignant change
- A molecular marker of disease, a quantitative assessment of the BCR/ABL transcripts in the blood is an excellent way or determining response and monitoring the effect of treatment
- Loss of the molecular response is usually the first sign that the patient is in danger of relapse of his/her disease

- The use of TKIs has dramatically altered the way patients with CML are treated
- Stem cell transplantation cures about 70% of patients but early mortality, infertility and chronic graft versus host disease remain major problems, therefore treatment with TKIs is always considered for initial therapy
- TKIs are very expensive so in some countries with limited health care resources stem cell transplantation is the first option

Further reading

Baccarani M, Saglio G, Goldman J, *et al.* Evolving concepts in the management of chronic myeloid leukemia: recommendations from an expert panel on behalf of the European Leukemia Net. *Blood* 2006; **108**: 1809–1820.

Carella AM, Daley GQ, Eaves CJ, Goldman JM & Hehlmann R, eds. *Chronic Myeloid Leukaemia: Biology and Treatment.* Martin Dunitz, 2001.

Sawyers CS. Chronic myeloid leukemia. *New England Journal of Medicine* 1999; **340**: 1330–1340.

Sawyers CL. Mechanisms of leukemogenesis. In: Stamatoyannopoulos G, Majerus PW, Perlmutter PM, Varmus H, eds. *The Molecular Basis of Blood Diseases*, 3rd edn. WB Saunders, 2001: 832–860.

Sawyers CL & Shah NP. Chronic myelogenous leukemia. In: Hoffman R, Benz EJ, Shatil SJ, Furie B, Cohen HJ, Silberstein LE, *et al.* eds. *Hematology: Basic Principles and Practice*, 4th edn. Churchill Livingstone, 2004: 1247–1253.

www.cancer.gov/cancerinfo/pdq/treatment/CML/patient/ Accessed in 2008.

www.ncbi.nlm.nih.gov/pubmed/16709930 Accessed in 2008.

A 62-year-old man who cannot button his shirt collar

John Snow is a 62-year-old Caucasian man who noticed a decrease in his energy over the last 2 weeks and a difficulty in buttoning his shirt collar because of a swelling in his neck. John had always been fit and energetic. He is a non-smoker and drinks only an occasional glass of wine at the weekend. John plays golf one afternoon per week.

What is your differential diagnosis?

The causes of a neck swelling that would make buttoning a collar difficult are quite limited. The swelling could be caused by the following:

1 An enlarged thyroid gland
2 Enlarged lymph nodes
3 A mass not related to any local anatomical structure, e.g. metastases from a cancer elsewhere
4 Obstruction of the superior vena cava, usually caused by a tumour in the anterior mediastinum
5 Inflammatory and/or infectious lesions in the mouth, throat or anywhere in the head and neck region

What should be done next?

Take a full history.

What are the important issues when taking the history?

The duration the symptoms have been present. Ask specific questions and link them to an event in his personal life or a public event. Ask about the severity of his fatigue. Has it interfered with his golf? Is the swelling in his neck painful and has it increased in size? When enquiring about night sweats ask if the patient changes his/her bed clothes or night attire.

Haematology: Clinical Cases Uncovered. By S. McCann, R. Foà, O. Smith and E. Conneally. Published 2009 by Blackwell Publishing, ISBN: 978-1-4051-8322-2

John had been at an important dinner in his golf club 4 months ago and had difficulty then with buttoning his shirt and tying his bow tie. For the past 2–3 months he played only 9 instead of 18 holes of golf.

The swelling has never been painful and he thinks that it is increasing in size.

Obstruction of the superior vena cava would usually be accompanied by a feeling of 'fullness' in the head and by a dusky blue appearance. A family history of thyroid disease is important as it may occur in more than one family member. Viral infections, e.g. infectious mononucleosis, can cause transient lymph node enlargement, but would be very uncommon in a patient of this age. Other symptoms such as weight loss and night sweats commonly occur in diseases such as Hodgkin's disease, non-Hodgkin's lymphoma and chronic lymphocytic leukaemia.

> **KEY POINT**
>
> Inflammatory (infectious) lesions are usually painful. Malignant swellings are commonly painless.

There was no family history of thyroid disease. John had never been ill before, apart from a fractured clavicle as a teenager. He has been married for 35 years and has two children aged 33 and 31 years of age who are both in good health.

What should be done next?

A physical examination.

John appeared well. His temperature was 37°C, blood pressure 125/75 mmHg. His mouth and throat appeared normal. He had enlarged lymph nodes in his cervical,

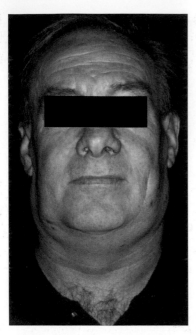

Figure 73 Enlarged lymph nodes in the neck.

Table 33 Results of the patient's full blood count and blood film (Fig. 74).

	Patient's results	Normal range
Hb	14.2 g/dL	13.5–18.0 g/dL
WBC	55.0 × 10⁹/L	4.0–11.00 × 10⁹/L (10³/µL)
Platelets	230 × 10⁹/L	140–450 × 10⁹/L (10³/µL)
Neutrophils	5.5 × 10⁹/L	2.0–7.5 × 10⁹/L (10³/µL)
Lymphocytes	49.5 × 10⁹/L	1.5–3.5 × 10⁹/L (10³/µL)

Hb, haemoglobin; WBC, white blood cell count.

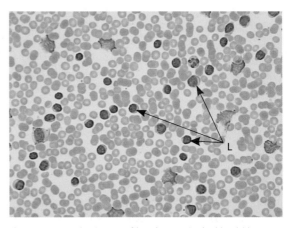

Figure 74 A predominance of lymphocytes in the blood (L).

submandibular and supraclavicular regions (3 × 2 cm; Fig. 73). They were non-tender, firm and fixed. The overlying skin appeared normal. The nodes in his axillae and groin were also enlarged (3 × 3 cm). John's spleen was palpable 5 cm below the left lower ribs.

Now what is your differential diagnosis?

Multiple enlarged lymph nodes, splenomegaly and fatigue are most likely caused by a haematological malignancy.

What should be done next?

A full blood count (Table 33), blood film (Fig. 74), biochemical screen, a chest radiograph and computed tomography (CT) scan of the thorax and abdomen (Fig. 75).

What should the patient be told?

He should be told that the diagnosis is not clear, but there is a significant possibility that he has a blood disease. He could continue to work but should return, with his wife/partner, for further discussion when the test results become available.

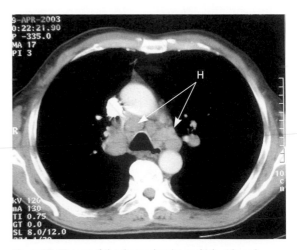

Figure 75 CT scan of the thorax showing multiple enlarged mediastinal lymph nodes (H).

How can the blood results be interpreted?

The lymphocyte count is elevated indicating an increased marrow output of lymphocytes. The most likely explanation for this in view of his age and physical findings is a chronic malignant lymphoproliferative disease.

The haemoglobin and platelet count are normal, therefore marrow function has been preserved.

In view of these findings, John should be referred to a haematologist.

What should the haematologist do next?

Interview John and repeat the history and physical examination. Examine the blood film and carry out a bone marrow aspirate and biopsy (Fig. 76).

The physical findings were confirmed and a detailed history revealed that the patient thought that an elderly uncle had died from some form of leukaemia.

What is the most likely diagnosis?

Chronic lymphocytic leukaemia (CLL).

Why is chronic lymphocytic leukaemia the most likely diagnosis?

The combination of a raised lymphocyte count, enlarged lymph nodes and spleen in a male patient

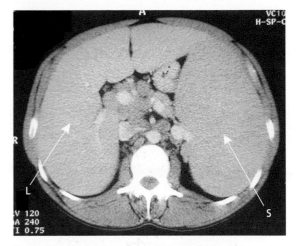

Figure 77 Computed tomography (CT) examination of the abdomen showing a large liver (L) and spleen (S).

aged 62 years are all typical findings in CLL. On examination of the blood film, most of the lymphocytes had the appearance of 'mature' lymphocytes and a number of cells with disrupted cytoplasm were seen (smear cells).

> **KEY POINT**
>
> There is an increased risk of CLL in first degree relatives of patients with CLL.

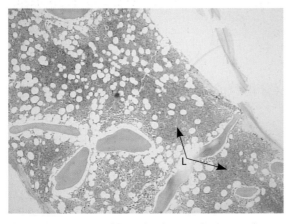

Figure 76 Bone marrow biopsy showing a predominance of lymphocytes (L).

The biochemical screen was normal. A CT scan of the thorax and abdomen (Fig. 77) showed enlarged lymph nodes, liver and spleen.

What other tests should be carried out to confirm the diagnosis?

Flow cytometry of the peripheral blood (Part 1). The lymphocyte population was made up almost entirely of B cells (normally T cells predominate in the blood). The B lymphocytes were 'clonal', i.e. they expressed immunoglobulin (Ig) on their cell surface with a single light chain only, κ or λ. Ig are characteristically expressed at low levels by CLL cells. The majority of lymphocytes expressed CD5 on their surface which is a typical finding in CLL.

Table 34 The patient's immunoglobulin (Ig) levels.

	Patient's results	Normal range
IgG	3.0 g/L (300 mg/dL)	6.26–14.96 g/L (700–1450 mg/dL)
IgA	0.17 g/L (17 mg/dL)	0.62–2.90 g/L (70–370 mg/dL)
IgM	0.13 g/L (13 mg/dL)	0.47–1.82 g/L (30–210 mg/dL)

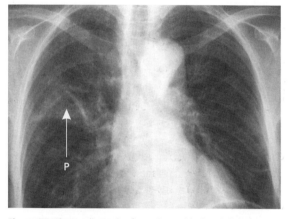

Figure 78 Chest radiograph of a patient with chronic lymphocytic leukaemia (CLL) with pneumonia (P).

> **KEY POINT**
>
> CLL is the most frequent leukaemia in the Western hemisphere. Although it usually occurs in the elderly (median age at presentation is 65 years), about 20% of patients are less than 55 years at the time of presentation. It occurs more frequently in men than women.

What further investigations should be carried out?

The serum levels of Ig (Table 34).

The cancer cells in CLL (as in most malignancies) are non-functional. Therefore, the levels of Ig in the patient's serum are frequently decreased (hypogammaglobulinaemia).

What infections occur in patients with hypogammaglobulinaemia?

These patients are prone to respiratory infections with Gram-positive encapsulated bacteria (Fig. 78).

> **KEY POINT**
>
> Opsonization is a process where Ig coat bacteria with 'complement' sequences leading to ingestion and killing by white cells (phagocytosis). This process is severely compromised in patients with CLL and hypogammaglobulinaemia.

What measures can be considered for patients with CLL and hypogammaglobulinaemia to reduce the risk of infection?

These patients should receive vaccination against *Streptococcus pneumoniae*, *Haemophilus influenzae* and influenza.

Why should patients with CLL and hypogammaglobulinaemia be vaccinated against the above infectious agents?

The impairment of Ig production (antibody synthesis) is not total and patients will demonstrate a partial response. Some antibody is made which clinically offers some protection from infection.

What other measures can reduce the risk of recurring chest infections?

Smoking cessation. If recurrent infections are a problem, replacement therapy with human pooled Ig should be commenced.

What are the dangers of giving blood products manufactured from many litres of human plasma?

There is a risk of transmitting HIV, hepatitis B or C, unknown viruses or prions.

> **KEY POINT**
>
> The risk is minimal with careful screening of the donors, meticulous testing of the plasma products and steps taken in the manufacturing process to inactivate or eliminate viruses.

What other types of infection occur frequently in patients with CLL?

Infections with herpes viruses causing 'cold sores' or herpes zoster (Fig. 79).

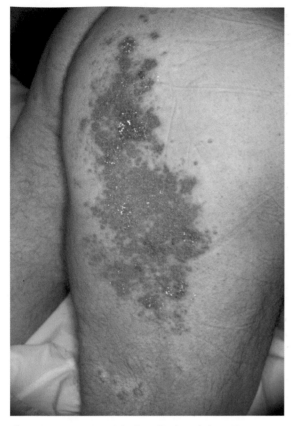

Figure 79 Herpes zoster infection affecting sciatic nerve distribution in a patient with CLL and hypogammaglobulinaemia.

KEY POINT

In spite of hypogammaglobulinaemia, patients with CLL may experience severe autoimmune haemolytic anaemia. This usually responds to treatment with steroids and does not influence survival.

What are the principles of treatment of patients with CLL?

Treatment is considered when there is evidence of disease progression. Symptoms such as night sweats, weight loss and fatigue, extensive lymph node enlargement, anaemia or a low platelet count because of bone marrow failure are all indications for treatment. More recently, combinations of chemotherapeutic agents and monoclonal antibodies are being explored. Many patients have a complete response to these combinations and we are unable to detect so-called minimal residual disease. Preliminary evidence suggests that these newer treatments will result in prolonged survival.

KEY POINT

Attempts are currently being made to 'stratify' patients at diagnosis in order to predict the risk of disease progression and requirement for treatment. Using techniques of flow cytometry and genetic analysis (fluorescence *in situ* hybridization; FISH) the following stratification can be used:

IgV$_H$	Mutated	Low risk
FISH	Normal or 13q-	
IgV$_H$	Mutated or	Intermediate risk
FISH	Trisomy 12	
IgV$_H$	Unmutated or	High risk
FISH	17p- or 11q-	

Can you construct an algorithm to help you to investigate a middle-aged man or woman with enlarged lymph nodes in his/her neck?

Yes.

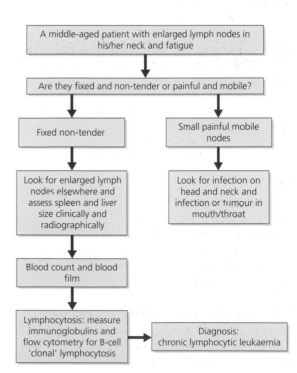

Outcome. John was treated with a combination of chemotherapy and antibodies to CLL cells and had an excellent response. He did not require Ig replacement therapy, but was vaccinated. John was advised to have 'cold sores' treated promptly and to contact his doctor immediately if he was in contact with an individual with chickenpox or shingles. He remained at work and was able to resume his 18 holes of golf weekly.

The following year his disease relapsed with a recurrence of symptoms and a rapidly rising white cell count. In spite of numerous combinations of chemotherapeutic agents and corticosteroids John died 6 months later from progressive disease.

CASE REVIEW

A 62-year-old man is concerned about his lack of energy and neck swelling. The swelling in his neck is clearly caused by lymph node enlargement and is part of a generalized picture of a large liver and spleen and widespread lymphadenopathy. The blood count and the examination of the blood film are diagnostic of chronic lymphocytic leukaemia.

Further tests are carried out to confirm the diagnosis and try to find some criteria that might influence prognosis. Thrombocytopaenia and anaemia from bone marrow failure indicate a poor outcome.

There are other forms of malignant lymphoproliferative disease such as non-Hodgkin's lymphoma and acute lymphoblastic leukaemia but the blood findings will be different.

This patient has active disease with symptoms and organomegaly. He is made aware of all the secondary problems particularly infections and how they can be prevented. This is as important as treating his leukaemia.

In spite of a good response to treatment his disease relapsed and proved fatal. There is still no cure for patients with CLL but the combinations of chemotherapy and rituximab (a monoclonal antibody against CD20 found on the surface of CLL lymphocytes) may be associated with complete remissions. This may be associated with better survival but evidence for cure must await longer follow-up.

KEY POINTS

- CLL is a common form of leukaemia
- Recent studies suggest that patients with chromosomal abnormalities such as 17p- of 11p- have a poor outlook and those with an isolated 13q- have a better survival
- B lymphocytes normally migrate to the germinal follicle of lymph nodes. Here they are exposed to various antigens and the immunoglobulin genes undergo somatic hypermutation (Part 1a). The B lymphocytes from patients with CLL may be hypermutated or not and this will influence the outcome as patients with the former have a better prognosis
- In patients with recurrent infections and hypogammaglobulinaemia human immunoglobulin replacement therapy is very effective
- Allogeneic stem cell transplantation may have a role in some young patients with aggressive disease
- There are two clinical staging systems: Rai and Binet, which help to indicate which patients require treatment
- Always examine a blood film before considering a lymph node biopsy and many patients will be spared this procedure

Further reading

Cheson BD, ed. *Chronic Lymphoid Leukemias*. Marcel Dekker, Inc., 2001.

Gentile M, Mauro FR, Guarini A & Foà R. New developments in the diagnosis, prognosis and treatment of chronic lymphocytic leukemia. *Current Opinion in Oncology* 2005; **17**: 597–604.

Hallek M, Cheson BD, Catovsky D, *et al*. Guidelines for the diagnosis and treatment of chronic lymphocytic leukemia: a report from the International Workshop on Chronic Lymphocytic Leukemia (IWCLL) updating the National Cancer Institute-Working Group (NCI-WG) 1996 guidelines. *Blood* 2008; **111**: 5446–5560.

Matutes E, Morilla R & Catovsky D. Immunophenotyping. In: Lewis SM, Bain BJ & Bates I, eds. *Dacie and Lewis: Practical Haematology*, 10th edn. Churchill Livingstone, 2006: 335–355.

Mauro FR, Foà R, Cerretti R, *et al*. Autoimmune haemolytic anemia in chronic lymphocytic leukaemia: clinical, therapeutic and prognostic features. *Blood* 2000; **95**: 2786–2792.

Shanfelt D, Byrd JC, Call TG, Zent CS & Kay NE. Narrative review: initial management of newly diagnosed, early stage chronic lymphocytic leukemia. *Annals of Internal Medicine* 2006; **145**: 453–447.

www.ncbi.nlm.nih.gov/pubmed/18216293 Accessed in 2008.

A 40-year-old man with fatigue and a sore throat

Bernard Grossman, a 40-year-old plumber, noticed a decrease in energy for a few weeks and has a sore throat for almost a week. He normally works 11 hours and often does emergency calls at weekends. Bernard goes hill walking at weekends but has not been able to do this for 3 weeks. He went to his family doctor because he had a sore throat, noticed a rash on his legs and he was bleeding from his gums for a few days, which frightened him.

What is your differential diagnosis?

The loss of energy and the pallor could be caused by anaemia. The petechial rash suggests an inflammation of the small blood vessels (vasculitis) or a reduced platelet count (thrombocytopenia). The sore throat, which was erythematous, suggests an infection.

The combination of these signs and symptoms suggests a bone marrow problem resulting in failure of the normal blood functions, i.e. anaemia, bleeding and infection.

What should be done next?

A physical examination.

Bernard appeared healthy but looked pale and had a petechial rash (purpura) on his legs (Fig. 80). His throat was red and inflamed. There was no lymphadenopathy and his spleen and liver were not enlarged. There were no fundal haemorrhages.

What is the meaning of purpura?

Purpura means bleeding into the skin. If it causes small pinpoint red spots they are known as 'petechiae' and if the bleeding becomes confluent it is called an 'ecchymosis'. To distinguish this from a dilated blood vessel

Haematology: Clinical Cases Uncovered. By S. McCann, R. Foà, O. Smith and E. Conneally. Published 2009 by Blackwell Publishing, ISBN: 978-1-4051-8322-2

gentle pressure is applied to the area. If bleeding has occurred into the skin (purpura) the lesion will not change colour. If the lesion is caused by a dilated blood vessel it will 'blanch' (lose its colour) and the red colour will return in a few seconds when the pressure is removed.

What investigations should be performed?

A full blood count (Table 35), blood film (Fig. 81) and biochemical screen (Table 36).

KEY POINT

He should be asked to wait for the results because of the probability of a serious underlying pathology.

The laboratory technician said that many of the lymphocytes looked like leukaemic 'blasts' but she wanted the haematologist to review the blood film. The platelet count was low. She suspected the patient had acute leukaemia (Fig. 81).

Now what is your differential diagnosis?

The sudden onset of symptoms together with anaemia and thrombocytopaenia could be a result of aplastic anaemia. However, the raised white cell count rules this out and using the information provided by the person examining the blood film a diagnosis of acute leukaemia is probable.

Acute infections such as infectious mononucleosis can produce abnormal white cells in the blood but you would not expect anaemia or thrombocytopaenia. Chronic lymphocytic leukaemia (CLL) can produces an elevated lymphocyte count but the appearances of the cells were

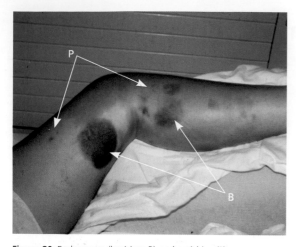

Figure 80 Ecchymoses (bruising; B) and petichiae (P).

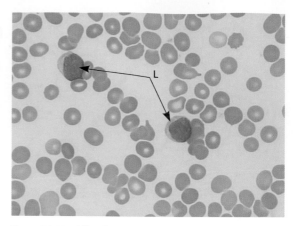

Figure 81 Blood film showing leukaemia blasts (L) showing no evidence of maturation.

Table 35 Results of full blood count.

	Patient's results	Normal range
Hb	9.0 g/dL	13.5–18.0 g/dL
MCV	87.0 fL	83.0–99.0 fL (µm³)
WBC	35.4 × 10⁹/L	4.0–11.0 × 10⁹/L (10³/µL)
Neutrophils	1.0 × 10⁹/L	2.0–7.5 × 10⁹/L (10³/µL)
Lymphocytes	34.4 × 10⁹/L	1.5–3.5 × 10⁹/L (10³/µL)
Platelets	20.0 × 10⁹/L	150–450 × 10⁹/L (10³/µL)

Hb, haemoglobin; MCV, mean corpuscular volume; WBC, white blood cell count.

Table 36 Results of the biochemical screen.

	Patient's results	Normal range
Creatinine	125 µmol/L	50–115 µmol/L (0.5–1.7 mg/dL)
Urate	600 µmol/L	150–470 µmol/L (3.0–8.0 mg/dL)
Lactic dehydrogenase	1000 IU/L	230–450 IU/L

Table 37 Lifespan of blood cells.

	Lifespan
Red cell	120 days
Neutrophil	4–6 hours
Lymphocyte	Years
Platelet	7–10 days

reported to be like 'leukaemic blasts', which would not be the appearance in CLL (Case 11).

Acute leukaemia can cause dramatic symptoms and signs within a few days or weeks.

What happens in acute leukaemia to produce these symptoms, signs and blood findings?

Normally, the bone marrow (the factory that produces the blood cells) produces red blood cells, white cells and platelets in a very orderly fashion so that the numbers of these cells in the blood remains relatively constant throughout life (Table 37).

KEY POINT

If the bone marrow fails to produce normal blood cells, the rate of reduction in the cell numbers in the blood will reflect the 'normal' lifespan of that cell. Clinically this means that a reduction in the number of neutrophils precedes the fall in platelets and red cells.

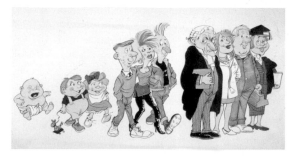

Figure 82 Normal maturation and function.

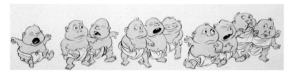

Figure 83 Simulation acute leukaemia where there is failure of maturation and function.

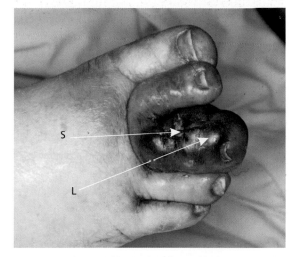

Figure 84 Leukaemic infiltration into the toe (L); the suture marks (S) are from the biopsy site.

What fundamental change is taking place in the bone marrow in acute leukaemia?

Leukaemic cells fail to differentiate (Figs 82 and 83), i.e. they fail to develop the normal function expected of them. They also have a reduced rate of apoptosis (programmed cell death).

Acquired genetic abnormalities which include gene translocations, deletions and mutations are the major mechanisms for failure of maturation and reduced rate of apoptosis. These genetic aberrations influence intracellular signalling, cell growth, differentiation and apoptotic rates. Leukaemia cells are called 'blasts'.

Why is the production of red cells and platelets in the marrow affected in leukaemia?

Leukaemia cells inhibit the development of normal cell differentiation in the non-involved cells in the bone marrow, probably by releasing cytokines.

How would you manage this patient?

Tell Bernard that he has a serious blood disease and arrange immediate admission to hospital.

Bernard was admitted to a specialist haematology unit. His history was verified. There was no known exposure to

marrow toxins or drugs that could cause these blood findings. The physical findings were confirmed and the optic fundi were examined for haemorrhage. His gums appeared hypertrophic (increase in gum tissue around the base of the teeth). His blood pressure was checked.

Why is it important to check the fundi?

A low platelet count can cause bleeding into the macula, which can cause blindness. Fresh bleeding in the fundi may predict bleeding into the brain and therefore needs immediate management.

Bernard's blood pressure was 125/75 mmHg (normal 120/80 mmHg).

KEY POINT

An elevated blood pressure together with a low platelet count increases the risk of intracerebral bleeding.

What is the relevance of the gum hypertrophy?

In some forms of leukaemia the leukaemic cells invade the gum tissue and cause it to swell. This is usually found in leukaemias of monocytic origin. Other tissues can also be invaded (Fig. 84).

What drugs should be specifically enquired about?

Bernard should be specifically asked about ingestion of aspirin or anti-inflammatory drugs within the preceding week. These drugs are in very common usage and people often forget that they have taken them.

KEY POINT

Aspirin does not influence the platelet count but may cause bleeding because of inhibition of platelet function. Aspirin and to a lesser extent non-steroidal anti-inflammatory drugs inhibit the cyclo-oxygenase pathway and interfere with platelet function. This reaction is not reversible and therefore platelet function will not recover until new platelets are released from the bone marrow.

What investigations should be performed next?

A bone marrow sample should be taken from the posterior iliac crest and sent to the laboratory for investigation. The blood count should be repeated with liver, bone and renal biochemical profiles (Table 36).

How can the abnormal biochemical findings be explained?

A high cell turnover will result in an elevated lactic dehydrogenase (LDH) and urate and cause renal impairment leading to a high creatinine level.

Bernard was given intravenous fluids to reduce the urate and creatinine levels and the nurses were instructed not to give any intramuscular injections (a low platelet count could cause severe bleeding). Allopurinol (a xanthine oxidase inhibitor) was given to reduce the urate level. A sample of urine was sent for microbiological analysis and a chest radiograph was carried out. Bernard was instructed about mouth care to minimize the risk of further infection. He was given broad-spectrum antibiotics because he was febrile (temperature 38.5°C). The urine did not contain any granulocytes and the chest radiograph was normal.

Why would you begin antibiotics before a diagnosis of infection is made?

Because patients with low granulocyte counts cannot mount the normal inflammatory response the usual signs of infection are commonly absent. Treatment with antibiotics should be given empirically for a presumed infection.

KEY POINT

The diagnosis of bacterial infection depends, to a large extent, on the signs of inflammation. Swelling, redness and pain are the common signs of infection because of the infecting organism and the granulocyte and monocyte response. Granulocytes in the urine or an infiltrate (shadow) on a chest radiograph are signs of infection in a normal individual.

Bernard was given a platelet transfusion and the site of the bone marrow aspiration was carefully monitored for bleeding.

The bone marrow examination confirmed a diagnosis of acute myeloid leukaemia (Fig. 85).

Why is it important to diagnose the specific type of leukaemia?

The type of leukaemia is important because it will influence the treatment and probable outcome.

Leukaemias are typed by trying to determine how the leukaemic cell would have developed under normal circumstances. Because the leukaemic cells are undifferentiated the morphology is not always conclusive in making a diagnosis of the type of leukaemia and a number of other investigations must be carried out.

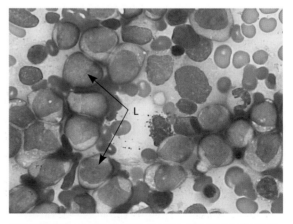

Figure 85 Bone marrow aspirate showing replacement of normal marrow with leukaemia blasts (L).

Table 38 Methods used to classify leukaemia.

Morphology	The appearance of the leukaemia cells on a glass slide (Fig. 81)
Cytochemistry	Special stains to try to identify primitive cell constituents, which might provide a clue as to the possible differentiation pathway that had been blocked in that cell
Flow cytometry	A study of the surface antigens on the leukaemic cell
Cytogenetics	Determination of the aberrant genetic material in the leukaemia cell (Fig. 86)
Molecular genetics	Study of the cDNA of the leukaemic cell. This is also useful to 'track' the patient after therapy to see if the leukaemia has been eradicated (Fig. 87).

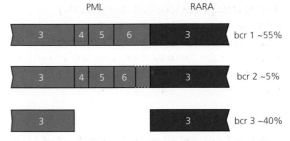

Figure 86 An illustration of a translocation between chromosomes 15 and 17 in acute promyelocytic leukaemia.

RT-PCR PML-RARα

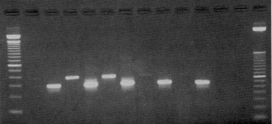

O = outer (1st round PCR),

N = nested (2nd round PCR), C3 = control –3 dilution,

C4 = control –4 dilution; -ve = negative control

Figure 87 A gel following reverse transcriptase polymerase chain reaction (RT-PCR) showing in lanes 1, 2 and 3 the abnormal 15:17 translocation in acute promyelocytic leukaemia. Lanes 1, 2 and 3 contain patient material. Lanes C3 and C4 are controls.

What further investigations will help to elucidate the diagnosis?

See Table 38 for further investigations to help the diagnosis.

The significance of the diagnosis was explained to Bernard and his wife and he was given combination chemotherapy.

How common is it to diagnose leukaemia in an adult?

The frequency is the same in adults and in children. Most adults with leukaemia are over the age of 50 years at the time of diagnosis.

The common cell of origin in adult leukaemia is myeloid (derived from granulocyte or monocyte precursor cells) and in children is lymphoid.

KEY POINT

In adults, the predominant form of leukaemia is myeloid, in which the leukaemic cells are of neutrophil and/or monocyte origin. Combination chemotherapy (anthracyclines being very important) results in a remission in most adults. Unfortunately, long-term survival is still around 50%. This is caused by relapsed disease or early death during induction chemotherapy from infection or bleeding.

What is the approach to treatment for myeloid leukaemias?

In general, combination chemotherapy is used for a number of cycles. Depending on the patient response and whether or not there are adverse prognostic factors (e.g. very high white cell count or specific genetic abnormalities), allogeneic stem cell transplantation will be considered. Stem cell transplantation is associated with a cure rate of over 60% but is complicated by graft versus host disease (GvHD) and infertility. Age is a major factor and young patients have a much better outcome.

Can you now construct an algorithm for a man with fatigue and sore throat?

Yes.

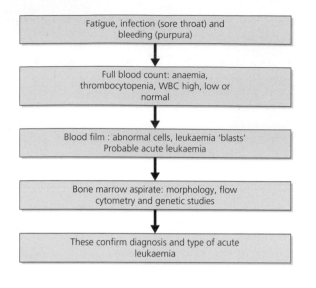

Fatigue, infection (sore throat) and bleeding (purpura)

↓

Full blood count: anaemia, thrombocytopenia, WBC high, low or normal

↓

Blood film : abnormal cells, leukaemia 'blasts' Probable acute leukaemia

↓

Bone marrow aspirate: morphology, flow cytometry and genetic studies

↓

These confirm diagnosis and type of acute leukaemia

Outcome. Bernard was treated with combination chemotherapy, which achieved a complete remission. He subsequently received three further courses of combination chemotherapy and proceeded to an allogeneic stem cell transplant from his human leucocyte antigen (HLA) identical sister. Bernard developed acute GvHD, which responded to treatment, and he is well and back at work 18 months after the transplant. Bernard remains in complete remission from his leukaemia.

CASE REVIEW

This man presented with the signs and symptoms of bone marrow failure. Correctly, a serious underlying haematological disease was suspected and he was referred to a specialist centre immediately. Examination of the blood film was critical in this case and the bone marrow findings confirmed the diagnosis. In most cases the onset of acute leukaemia is abrupt but occasionally it can be smouldering.

Signs of acute leukaemia are often confined to anaemia, bleeding and infection. Because of the low neutrophil level the usual signs of infection may be absent and fever may be the only clue.

The reasons for a rapid referral to a specialist unit are good support and care with treatment of infections, bleeding and anaemia and an accurate diagnosis of the type of leukaemia. Accurate diagnosis allows the haematologist to advise the most appropriate treatment and to discuss the advisability of stem cell transplantation. The details of the type of treatment offered and the role of stem cell transplantation are matters for a specialist.

KEY POINTS

- Acute leukaemia is a rare disease with an incidence of about 2 : 100,000 but increasing with age. It is not unusual to see a patient present in the sixth or seventh decade
- In the vast majority of cases the cause of the leukaemia is unknown. High doses of ionizing radiation (as in Japan during the Second World War) cause acute and chronic leukaemia but this is not relevant in the majority of cases
- Genetic abnormalities are present in most leukaemia cells but their precise role in causing the cells to behave in a malignant fashion is unknown

- In most cases the disease is sporadic but some families have more than one person with the disease. Presumably these families carry a genetic predisposition and are prone to leukaemia if they are exposed to the leukaemogenic agent
- The decision on the type of treatment offered and the role of stem cell transplantation depends on a number of prognostic indicators. These are continually under evaluation. The white cell count at diagnosis, the age of the patient and the type of genetic abnormality all influence the response to treatment and outcome
- The overall cure rate is about 50%

Further reading

Degos L, Linch D & Löwenberg B, eds. *Textbook of Malignant Haematology*. Martin Dunitz, 1999: 743–769.

Henderson E, Lister TA & Greaves MF. *Leukaemia*, 7th edn. Saunders, 2002.

Hoffbrand AV, Moss PAH & Pettit JE. *Essential Haematology*, 5th edn. Blackwell Science, Oxford, 2006: 157–173

Lowenberg B, Downing JR & Burnett A. Acute myeloid leukemia. *New England Journal of Medicine* 1999; **341**: 1051–1062.

McCormack E, Bruserud O & Gjertsen BT. Review: genetic models of acute myeloid leukaemia. *Oncogene* 2008; **27**: 3765–3779

www.ncbi.nlm.nih.gov/pubmed/18264136 Accessed in 2008.

www.cancer.gov/cancertopics/pdq/treatment/adultAML/ patient Accessed in 2008.

www.bcshguidelines.com/pdf/CLH135.PDF Accessed in 2006.

Case 13 A 58-year-old farmer with a broken rib

Francesco Sabattini, a 58-year-old farmer, stumbled and fell while herding his sheep. He complained of severe rib pain. His wife put him to bed and gave him aspirin. He had difficulty sleeping because of the pain so the next day they attended the family doctor's surgery.

The family doctor had known Francesco for many years. As well as the pain in his ribs his wife told the doctor that her husband had been complaining of low back pain for about 6 months. Francesco volunteered that he felt very tired at the end of the day and often 'nodded off' to sleep in a chair after his evening meal.

The doctor remarked that he thought Francesco 'looked a little smaller' than when he had seen him a few months earlier. He also thought Francesco looked a little pale.

What is your differential diagnosis?

Fatigue is difficult to evaluate and in this age group it could be caused by heart failure, anaemia or cancer. Depression is a common cause of fatigue. Arthritis would explain his back pain but is unlikely to make him pale. He may have an underlying neoplasm. The loss of height may suggest osteoporosis and collapse of a vertebral body.

The combination of back pain and pallor suggests a bone marrow problem.

The family doctor recommended radiographs of his back and ribs. Because Francesco was very busy he delayed going for the radiographs. A few weeks later he began to complain of nausea and shortness of breath. He developed a cough, which caused severe rib pain.

How does this information help with the differential diagnosis?

He has a cough and shortness of breath so this suggests a chest infection. The cough was making his rib pain worse because of the movement of the rib cage during breathing and coughing. A simple chest infection would not explain the rib pain, or the nausea. These symptoms together with the loss of height are indicative of a serious underlying problem.

The family doctor was quite worried and referred him to the local accident and emergency department.

What would the doctor on duty do first?

Take a history about previous illness, especially chest infections, smoking habit, alcohol consumption and medications.

Francesco had been very well until this episode. He had two chest infections in the last 6 months, which required treatment with antibiotics, which was unusual for him. He had smoked 20 cigarettes a day for all his adult life and had a glass of whiskey before retiring to bed. He drank 4–5 glasses of wine at weekends. He denied coughing blood and had not experienced hoarseness or any change in his voice. This information was verified by his wife.

Now what is your differential diagnosis?

Lung cancer is a definite possibility. His smoking history and recent chest infections are suspicious findings. Back pain could be a result of metastases from lung cancer. Lung cancer could also explain his pallor, as it may be associated with anaemia. Multiple myeloma can cause bone pain, anaemia and loss of height. The nausea is hard to explain but perhaps it was caused by the analgesics. An infection such as tuberculosis B could present as pneumonia and be associated with anaemia and bone pain.

On examination, Francesco's pulse was 120 beats/minute. His blood pressure is 120/60 mmHg and he had a fever of 38°C. He was pale and dehydrated. He had a marked

Haematology: Clinical Cases Uncovered. By S. McCann, R. Foà, O. Smith and E. Conneally. Published 2009 by Blackwell Publishing, ISBN: 978-1-4051-8322-2

kyphosis and there was decreased air entry with coarse crackles at the left lung base.

What investigations should be ordered?

A full blood count (Table 39), blood film (Fig. 88), renal, liver and bone profiles (Table 40).

I *The blood film (Fig. 88) showed 'rouleaux' formation.*

Now what is your differential diagnosis?

Francesco is anaemic and the 'rouleaux' formation of the red cells reflects an elevation of plasma fibrinogen or immunoglobulins. Fibrinogen is an acute-phase reactant and elevation suggests cancer or an inflammatory and/or infectious disease.

Table 39 Results of the full blood count.

	Patient's results	Normal range
Hb	8.5 g/dL	13.5–18.0 g/dL
MCV	90.0 fL	83.0–99.0 fL (μm^3)
White cell count	11.6×10^9/L	$4.0–11.0 \times 10^9$/L (10^3/μL)
Platelet count	160×10^9/L	$140–450 \times 10^9$/L (10^3/μL)
Differential white cell count	Normal	

Hb, haemoglobin; MCV, mean corpuscular volume.

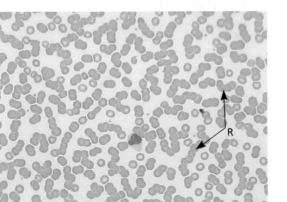

Figure 88 Blood film showing rouleaux formation (R).

> ### KEY POINT
>
> 'Rouleaux' formation means that the red cells appear like coins stacked upon each other. This happens because the red cells are covered with fibrinogen or immunoglobulin, which inhibits the charge that usually makes red cells repel each other.

What are the major abnormalities in the biochemistry profile?

The blood levels of calcium and creatinine are elevated. The total protein level is elevated and the albumin level is decreased.

Do these findings help in the differential diagnosis?

The elevated creatinine suggests renal failure, which could be caused by the hypercalcemia. The increased total protein and the low albumin suggest a disturbance of liver function.

The chest radiograph shows that Francesco has a left-sided pneumonia. In addition, he has a fractured rib (Fig. 89) and a multiple 'lytic' lesion in the humerus (Fig. 90). His lumbar spine shows evidence of osteoporosis (decrease in mineralization) and collapse of a number of vertebrae.

The vertebral collapse has led to the kyphosis. The combination of rouleaux formation in the blood film, pneumonia and lytic lesions in the bones is strong evidence for multiple myeloma.

Table 40 Results of the biochemical screen.

	Patient's results	Normal range
Serum creatinine	215.0 mmol/L	50–115 mmol/l (0.5-1.7 mg/dL)
Calcium	3.36 mmol/L	2.20–2.70 mmol/L (8.6–10.3 mg/dL)
Albumin	26.0 g/L	35–50 g/L (3.5–5.0 g/dL)
Total protein	95.5 g/L	60–80 g/L (6.0–8.0 g/dL)

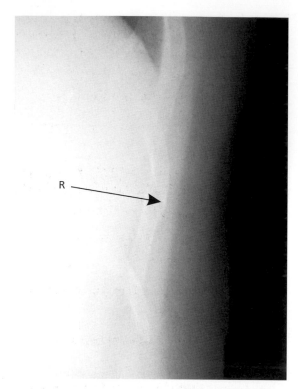

Figure 89 A localized view showing a fractured rib (R).

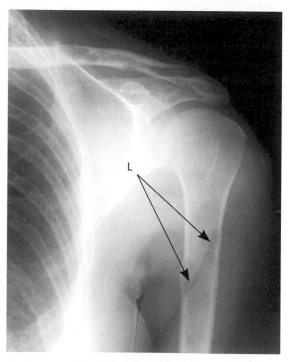

Figure 90 A radiograph showing multiple lytic lesions in the humerus (L).

> **KEY POINT**
>
> Some cancers produce cytokines, which can cause resorption of bone (osteolytic activity) or cytokines that induce the proliferation of osteoblasts (osteoblastic activity), which are the cells responsible for new bone formation. Cytokines are soluble proteins produced by a wide variety of haematopoietic and non-haematopoietic cells. Pathological fractures are fractures that occur at sites of osteolytic bone lesions.

When would a radionucleotide bone scan be preferable?

Radionucleotide scans are very informative when osteoblastic lesions are being investigated. Osteolytic lesions are best detected by plain radiography or magnetic resonance imaging (MRI) (see Fig. 91).

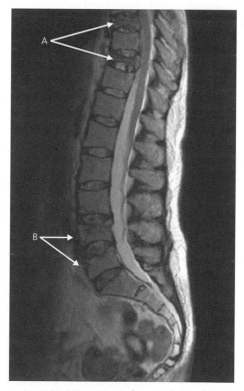

Figure 91 Pathological compression fractures of T8 and T10 (A) vertebral bodies, in a patient with multiple myeloma. Note, in addition, fractures of the superior end plates of L4 and L5 (B).

Which tumours frequently give rise to bone lesions?

Bone metastasis from cancer of the:

1 Prostate
2 Breast
3 Lung
4 Kidney
5 Bladder
6 Thyroid

These lesions are usually osteoblastic. Metastatic tumours to bone are much more common than primary bone tumours.

Multiple myeloma causes osteolytic lesions of bone.

What other blood tests should be performed to confirm your suspicions?

Measurement of serum immunoglobulins (Table 41).

What cells normally produce immunoglobulin and what does the term 'monoclonal band' mean?

B lymphocytes normally produce immunoglobulins (antibodies), which bind foreign antigens, e.g. bacteria and viruses. Immunoglobulins represent the output of millions of different plasma cells. The normal response consists of molecules of immunoglobulins with different mixtures of κ and λ light chains. A monoclonal (M) band reflects the synthesis of immunoglobulin (Ig) from a single clone of plasma cells and, therefore, one light chain type. These monoclonal proteins are called 'paraproteins'.

Table 41 Immunoglobulin levels in the patient's blood.

Serum immunoglobulins*	Patient's results	Normal range (male)
IgG	66.0 g/L (6600 mg/dL)	6.40–15.22 g/L (700–1450 mg/dL)
IgA	0.20 g/L (20 mg/dL)	0.48–3.44 g/L (70–370 mg/dL)
IgM	0.15 g/L (15 mg/dL)	0.29–1.86 g/L (30–210 mg/dL)

*In normal individuals immunoglobulins are polyclonal, i.e. have a mixture of λ and κ light chains.

What do these results suggest?

A raised IgG level and reduced IgA and IgM levels in Francesco's blood suggest a disease affecting B cells, most likely multiple myeloma.

What further blood tests should be performed?

Electrophoresis of the serum proteins (Figs 92, 93).

KEY POINT

In multiple myeloma the monoclonal band is most commonly IgG (60%).

What other test should be performed to prove monoclonality?

Immunofixation of the serum.

Antibodies to IgG, IgA, IgM, κ and λ are used to show the protein has a single light chain.

What is the significance of the low IgA and IgM?

Most cancer cells are non-functional. In multiple myeloma the abnormal B cells produce a monoclonal non-functional protein and also fail to produce a normal antibody response. Therefore, the patient has

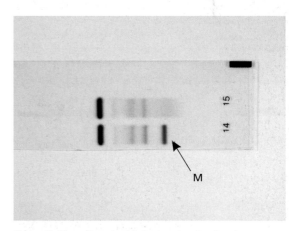

Figure 92 Electrophoresis of the serum proteins. Proteins are placed on a supporting matrix and separated according to size and charge. The dense staining in the immunoglobulin region suggests that there is a monoclonal protein present (M).

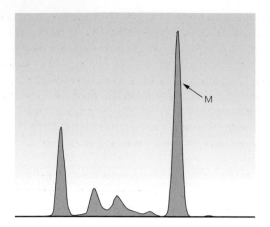

Figure 93 Densitometery scan of the serum proteins. M, monoclonal band.

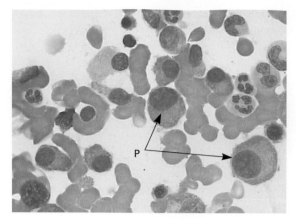

Figure 94 A bone marrow aspirate showing multiple malignant plasma cells (P) with dark blue cytoplasm and eccentric nucleus. The blue staining cytoplasm indicates immunoglobulin synthesis.

hypogammaglobulinaemia (a low level of immunoglobulins). This explains the low IgA and IgM. The low levels of immunoglobulins cause increased susceptibility to infection, which is the presenting feature in approximately 25% of patients with multiple myeloma.

KEY POINT

Patients with hypogammaglobulaemia are most prone to infections with encapsulated bacterial organisms. These patients have very poor antibody responses, especially to polysaccharide antigens such as those in the bacterial cell walls. The absence of antibodies directed against the bacterial capsule limits the ability of phagocytic cells to ingest and kill the bacteria. The most common infections in people with hypogammaglobulaemia are caused by *Streptococcus pneumoniae* or *Haemophilus influenzae*.

What other investigations should be performed to complete the diagnosis?

Bone marrow aspirate (Fig. 94) and β_2-microglobulin levels.

The combination of blood, marrow, biochemical and immunological findings confirms a diagnosis of multiple myeloma.

KEY POINT

Serum β_2-microglobulin (β_2-M) was raised at 3.0 mg/L (normal 1.05–2.05 mg/L). This is the single most powerful predictor of survival in patients with multiple myeloma.

What is β_2-microglobulin and is there any biological understanding of its importance?

β_2-M is the light chain gene of the class 1 histocompatibility antigen and is expressed on the surface of all nucleated cells. The increase in β_2-M in multiple myeloma is a reflection of the tumour mass. It is excreted by the kidneys and is also elevated in renal failure.

Renal failure occurs in about 25% of patients with multiple myeloma.

Besides morphological evaluation of the bone marrow what other investigations might be helpful?

A cytogenetic and molecular evaluation might be useful to confirm the diagnosis and provide some prognostic information.

What other radiological investigation is useful in establishing the extent of myeloma involvement?

An MRI (Fig. 91).

What else could the detection of a 'monoclonal' protein imply?

A monoclonal gammopathy of uncertain significance (MGUS). Patients with MGUS usually have a relatively low paraprotein. They have a normal haemoglobin and renal function. Ten per cent of the population over the age of 70 have MGUS. Because these patients are elderly the finding of a paraprotein usually occurs incidentally as part of a wider investigation of an unrelated illness. No treatment is indicated for MGUS but follow-up is necessary, as approximately 10% of patients with MGUS will ultimately develop multiple myeloma.

KEY POINT

Cells from the bone marrow in patients with MGUS contain many of the abnormalities seen in patients with multiple myeloma. The slow progression (1% per year) adds belief to the possibility of a 'second hit' occurring to trigger the malignant transformation to multiple myeloma. The nature of the 'second hit' remains unknown.

Because of the age of onset of MGUS there are other competing causes of death which reduces the risk of developing multiple myeloma from 25% in a patient of 50 years over a 25-year period to approximately 10%.

Can you construct an algorithm for the investigation of a patient with bone pain and anaemia?

Yes.

Recurrent infection, bone pain and anaemia

↓

Blood film Rouleaux formation

↓

Plain radiographs – osteopenia ± collapse of vertebrae MRI shows extent of MM involvement

↓

Renal, bone and liver profile Elevated β_2-microglobulin

↓

Serum immuno-electrophoresis

↓

Bone marrow aspirate and biopsy +/− Cytogenetic and molecular evaluation

Outcome. Francesco was admitted to hospital. His was given intravenous fluids to relieve his dehydration, hypercalcaemia and renal failure. In addition, Francesco was treated with a combination of corticosteroids and a bisphosphonate for the hypercalcaemia. He also received intravenous antibiotics for his chest infection and analgesia for his bone pain. Over the next few days Francesco's condition markedly improved with normalization of his creatinine and calcium. He was given chemotherapy followed by an autologous stem cell transplant.

One year later he is feeling very well and doing a full day's work on the farm. He no longer has any bone pain. His most recent immunoglobulins show that his paraprotein is no longer detectable.

On his last clinic visit he was delighted to tell you that 'Lydia, the cow' won first prize at his local agricultural show.

CASE REVIEW

This 58-year-old man presented with bone pain, suggestive of a rib fracture after minor trauma. The fact that the trauma was minor should alert you that something serious might be going on. Although his doctor was worried especially at the loss of height, the patient failed to attend for a radiograph. Women are much better at attending doctors and presenting for examinations than men. This may or may not be related to their experience with pregnancy and childbirth.

A careful history and physical examination suggested cancer and infection but the biochemical and marrow findings were diagnostic. The rouleaux formation on the blood film was an early clue and the immunoglobulin screen was very suggestive of myeloma.

It is very important to attend to the medical treatment of the patient including his infection, metabolic abnormalities and to provide adequate pain relief with narcotic analgesics. Pain relief is paramount as it facilitates mobilization and therefore reduces the progression of osteopenia.

KEY POINTS

- Recently, the treatment for multiple myeloma has become much more effective and myeloma has become a 'chronic disease' in many patients
- Thalidomide, a notorious anti-emetic which caused severe birth defects, and its successor lenalidomide are both very effective agents. Both are anti-angiogenic (inhibit the formation of new blood vessels) and down-regulate the production of TNFα but their precise mode of action in myeloma is unknown
- Proteasome inhibitors such as bortezomib which induce apoptosis (programmed cell death) in plasma cells are proving very effective

- The uses of combinations of the above drugs with corticosteroids produce a very favourable response in many patients. Patients who respond well are offered autologous stem cell transplantation with cells harvested when the patient has minimal disease. Although not curative this treatment often results in prolonged disease remission
- The medical management of the complications of myeloma are as important as the specific treatment of the disease

---

Further reading

http://asheducationbook.hematologylibrary.org/cgi/content/full/2005/1/340

Kyle RA, Morie MD, Gertz A, *et al*. Review of 1027 patients with newly diagnosed multiple myeloma. *Mayo Clinic Proceedings* 2003; **78**: 21–33.

National Cancer Institute. Multilple myeloma and other plasma cell neoplasms. www.cancer.gov/cancerinfo/pdq/treatment/myeloma/healthprofessional Accessed in 2008.

Trpos E, Politu M & Rahemtulla A. New insights into the pathophysiology and management of bone disease in multiple myeloma. *British Journal of Haematology* 2003; **123**: 758–769.

www.mayoclinic.com/health/multiple-myeloma/DS00415

Case 14 — An 18-year-old medical student who complained of bone pain following alcohol ingestion and a swelling on the right side of her neck

Sylvia Le Roy, an 18-year-old medical student, presented to the haematology clinic with a 4-week history of fatigue and general malaise. She had been to her family doctor on two occasions during this period for a sore throat for which she received antibiotics. Sylvia had noticed a swelling on the right side of her neck about 3 weeks ago.

What could be causing these symptoms?

Recurrent sore throat in a young person with fever and swelling in the neck suggests a viral infection. However, the degree of fatigue and malaise should make you suspicious of a more serious underlying disease such as a lymphoma.

What is your differential diagnosis?

Infectious mononucleosis, cytomegalovirus (CMV) infection, HIV primary infection, hepatitis A or B, rubella, adenovirus, toxoplasma infection, β-haemolytic streptococcal infection, a malignant lymphoma.

What should be done next?

A full history should be taken with emphasis on weight loss, anorexia, fever or night sweats, known as B symptoms. Any change in size of the swelling, pain or tenderness should be enquired about.

Sylvia admitted to a weight loss of 4 kg and night sweats on six occasions during the last month. The swelling had increased in size, but was never painful and was not tender to touch. She had an unproductive cough for 4 days. She had mild asthma for which she took bronchodilators with good effect. Sylvia noticed bone pain on a few occasions after consuming alcohol. There was no other history apart from the usual childhood illnesses.

Haematology: Clinical Cases Uncovered. By S. McCann, R. Foà, O. Smith and E. Conneally. Published 2009 by Blackwell Publishing, ISBN: 978-1-4051-8322-2

What is the significance of the night sweats, weight loss and bone pain induced by alcohol?

They are highly suggestive of non-Hodgkin's lymphoma or Hodgkin's disease. Although fever, sore throat and malaise can be found in a viral infection such as infectious mononucleosis, bone pain induced by alcohol, although rare, is a finding that appears to be specific to patients with Hodgkin's lymphoma.

What should be done next?

A full physical examination.

On examination, Sylvia was pale and appeared unwell. She had a mass in the right supraclavicular area (which measured 2 × 2 cm, was non-tender and fixed). There were no other enlarged lymph nodes and her liver and spleen were not enlarged. Sylvia had a temperature of 38°C.

What do the physical findings suggest?

Swellings in the supraclavicular area (usually lymph nodes) are almost invariably pathological. The pallor suggests anaemia and the fixed non-tender mass suggests a malignancy.

What type of anaemia would be most common in a girl of this age?

Iron deficiency anaemia would be the most common. The anaemia of chronic disease is a possibility especially in view of the likelihood of an underlying lymphoid malignancy.

What questions should be asked if iron deficiency is suspected?

A full dietary history, details of menstrual blood loss and any other evidence of bleeding.

A low iron intake is common in adolescence and can contribute to iron deficiency. Bleeding, particularly menorrhagia, is also a common cause of iron deficiency in this age group.

What is the significance of the fever?

A viral infection or an upper respiratory tract bacterial infection could cause a fever (she has a history of asthma and complained of an unproductive cough); however, fever can be a manifestation of lymphoproliferative diseases (B symptoms).

What investigations should be carried out?

A full blood count (Table 42), a blood film, biochemical screen (Table 43), erythrocyte sedimentation rate (ESR), viral screen, a chest radiograph and analysis of the sputum for evidence of infection.

The ESR was 60 mm/hour (normal female 0–15 mm/hour). The blood film showed an increased number of platelets, but no other abnormalities.

What blood film abnormalities would you expect to see in infectious mononucleosis?

The presence of atypical mononuclear cells (Fig. 95). The serology would be positive with immunoglobulin M (IgM) antibodies to the virus capsid antigen (VCA). This is an IgM antibody which appears during the acute infection and persists for a number of months. Epstein–Barr nuclear antigen (EBNA) develops after the acute illness and persists for life.

What could be the cause of the high platelet count?

An increased platelet count is commonly found in response to acute haemorrhage. It can also be found in malignancies and may be a manifestation of myeloproliferative diseases, e.g. chronic myeloid leukaemia (Case 10), polycythaemia rubra vera (Case 16) or iron deficiency (Case 1).

What is the significance of the elevated ESR?

The elevation is a non-specific finding in infections or malignancies.

Table 42 Results of the full blood count.

	Patient's results	Normal values (female)
Hb	8.3 g/dL	11.5–16.4 g/dL
MCV	69 fL	83–99 fL (μm^3)
WBC	8.1×10^9/L	$4–11 \times 10^9$/L (10^3/μL)
Neutrophils	5.4×10^9/L	$2–7.5 \times 10^9$/L (10^3/μL)
Lymphocytes	2.7×10^9/L	$1.5–3.5 \times 10^9$/L (10^3/μL)
Platelets	746×10^9/L	$140–450 \times 10^9$/L (10^3/μL)
Reticulocytes	85×10^9/L	$50–100 \times 10^9$/L (0.5–15%)

Hb, haemoglobin; MCV, mean corpuscular volume; WBC, white blood cell count.

Table 43 Biochemical screen.

	Patient's results	Normal values
Bilirubin	5 μmol/L	0–17 μmol/L (0.3–1.1 mg/dL)
Alkaline phosphatase	376 IU/L	40–120 IU/L
GGT	100 IU/L	5–40 IU/L
LDH	240 IU/L	230–450 IU/L
Ferritin	150 μg/L	20–300 μg/L (20–300 ng/mL)

GGT, gamma glutamyl transferase; LDH, lactic dehydrogenase.

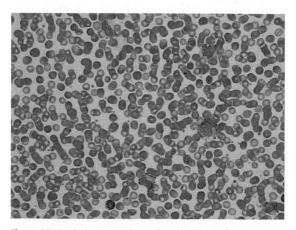

Figure 95 Atypical mononuclear cells in the blood of a patient with infectious mononucleosis.

The ESR measures the rate of sedimentation of red cells in a tube. Red cells are normally kept apart by van der Waal's forces. In patients with infection or malignancies, high levels of immunoglobulin (antibodies) or fibrinogen (a plasma coagulation protein) can inhibit these forces, allowing the red cells to stick together.

What test would you carry out to elucidate the mechanism of the raised ESR?

Serum protein electrophoresis and a coagulation screen.

The serum protein electrophoresis shows a polyclonal gammopathy. This indicates a normal response to infection, but can be a non-specific finding in malignancy. The coagulation screen revealed a fibrinogen of 12 g/L (normal 1.5–4.0 g/L), which explains the raised ESR. The synthesis of fibrinogen may be increased in malignancies.

The viral screen including EBV serology was negative excluding a diagnosis of infectious mononucleosis.

The chest radiograph (Fig. 96) showed enlargement of the right paratracheal nodes.

Now what is your differential diagnosis?

Sylvia is anaemic with a low MCV suggesting iron deficiency or the anaemia of chronic disease. The serum ferritin of 150 µg/L excludes iron deficiency. The high platelet count could be associated with a malignancy as there is no clinical evidence of acute haemorrhage. Sylvia's liver blood tests are abnormal suggesting a viral infection or malignancy. The chest radiograph confirms enlarged lymph nodes in the neck and upper mediastinum. These results together with her symptoms suggest a malignant lymphoproliferative disease including Hodgkin's lymphoma, non-Hodgkin's lymphoma or acute lymphoblastic leukaemia. Sarcoidosis could also present with hilar lymphadenopathy.

> **KEY POINT**
>
> Fever, night sweats and weight loss are known as B symptoms and are commonly found in Hodgkin's lymphoma, non-Hodgkin's lymphoma and chronic lymphocytic leukaemia.

How should this patient be managed?

Sylvia should be referred immediately to hospital for further investigation.

What further investigations should be carried out in the hospital?

A bone marrow aspirate and biopsy (Fig. 97) and a computed tomography (CT) scan of thorax and abdomen.

The bone marrow aspirate and biopsy showed increased iron stores in keeping with the diagnosis anaemia of chronic disease. The CT of thorax and abdomen showed adenopathy in the anterior mediastinum (Fig. 98).

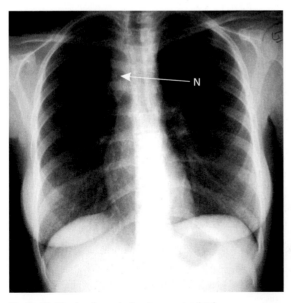

Figure 96 Chest radiograph showing paratracheal lymphadenopathy (N).

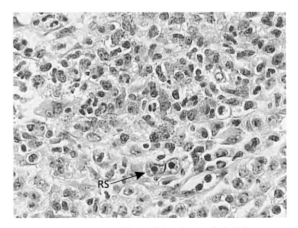

Figure 97 Bone marrow with Reed–Sternberg cells (RS) (i.e. Hodgkin's lymphoma).

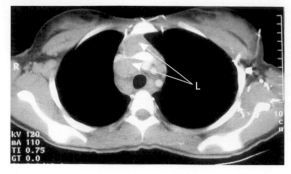

Figure 98 Computed tomography (CT) of thorax showing lymphadenopathy in the superior mediastinum (L).

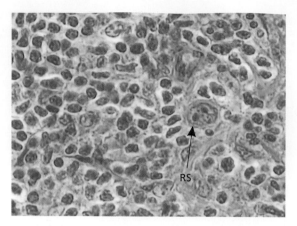

Figure 99 Lymph node biopsy shows Reed–Sternberg (RS) cells and collagen bands: nodular sclerosing Hodgkin's lymphoma.

> **KEY POINT**
>
> Bone marrow involvement in Hodgkin's lymphoma (Fig. 97) is extremely uncommon and occurs in less than 5% of patients. Marrow involvement significantly worsens the prognosis. Marrow involvement is extremely common in non-Hodgkin's lymphoma and does not have the same prognostic significance as in Hodgkin's disease.

> **KEY POINT**
>
> Hodgkin's lymphoma is most frequently seen in adolescents and young adults, but there is a second peak after the age of 50 years.

How do the investigations influence the management?

The extent of the disease will influence the type of management.

What are the principles of management of Hodgkin's lymphoma?

Hodgkin's lymphoma has been one of the earliest malignancies to be cured by combination chemotherapy. However, extensive nodal disease may also require radiotherapy.

The anaemia of chronic disease is characterized by a low MCV, but normal ferritin and bone marrow iron stores. It is commonly seen in association with malignancy or chronic infectious diseases such as tuberculosis. Hepsidin synthesis is increased in the anaemia of chronic disease and inhibits the escape of iron from macrophages thereby limiting its availability to form haem.

What should be done next?

A lymph node biopsy.

> **KEY POINT**
>
> The long-term cure rate for Hodgkin's lymphoma is now so good that the emphasis is being placed on limiting the toxicity of therapy.

A lymph node excision biopsy reveals nodular sclerosing Hodgkin's disease (Fig. 99).

Hodgkin's lymphoma is a malignancy most commonly of B-cell origin. It is manifested by enlarged lymph nodes, hepatosplenomegaly and B symptoms. The classic cell associated with Hodgkin's lymphoma is the Reed–Sternberg cell. There is evidence of EBV infection in many patients with Hodgkin's lymphoma, but a direct causative role has not been demonstrated.

Can you now construct an algorithm for a young patient with fever, night sweats and lymphadenopathy?

Yes.

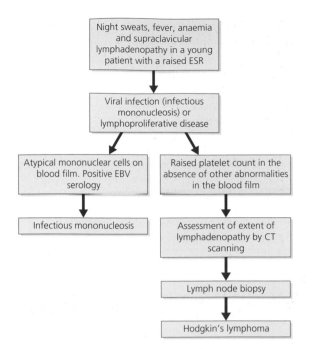

Outcome. Sylvia was treated with combination chemotherapy to which she had a complete response. She returned to her medical studies 6 months from the time of her diagnosis. Sylvia is currently a senior house officer in a large teaching hospital and remains in complete remission from her disease.

CASE REVIEW

A young girl presents to the doctor with a history of fatigue, malaise, weight loss and a sore throat. The most common diagnosis would be a fairly innocuous viral infection. Many patients with malignant lymphomas, Hodgkin's lymphoma or acute leukaemia are initially diagnosed incorrectly because these diseases are rare compared with common viral infections, such as infectious mononucleosis, adenovirus infections or even streptococcal throat infection.

What makes you suspicious is the persistence of symptoms and signs, and the marked degree of malaise, fatigue and weight loss. The presence of lymphadenopathy in the neck of a young person is always difficult as it may be associated with localized infection; in this case it is described in the supraclavicular area which is always pathological. The size of the node, the site and the fact that it is not painful and fixed suggest something more serious. The presence of anaemia would be unusual in a girl of this age unless it was totally unconnected, such as an iron deficiency resulting from menorrhagia. Anemia should make you suspicious of a systemic disorder in association with the symptoms and signs of sore throat, malaise, weight loss and lymphadenopathy.

The abnormal chest radiograph with the paratracheal lymphadenopathy is suggestive of a malignant process and taken together with the symptoms and signs warrants a lymph node excision biopsy. Further radiographical examination confirmed lymphadenopathy in the superior mediastinum and excision lymph node biopsy revealed a diagnosis of Hodgkin's lymphoma.

It is important that an excision lymph node biopsy is carried out by an experienced surgeon. Small lymph nodes that surround Hodgkin's lymphoma may reveal a reactive pattern only. Inexperienced doctors may, in their attempts to minimize surgery, remove small satellite nodes thereby giving a misleading diagnosis. In this case the correct procedure was carried out and a diagnosis was made confidently. The patient was then started on treatment. With current management the majority of these patients become long-term survivors.

KEY POINTS

- The presence of B symptoms together with persistent signs, symptoms, lymphadenopathy and weight loss alerts one to the suspicion of a malignant lymphoma
- In this age group, Hodgkin's lymphoma must be suspected although non-Hodgkin's lymphoma and acute lymphocytic leukaemia can also occur
- The relationship between EBV infection and Hodgkin's lymphoma is difficult to unravel. Epidemiology suggests that 50% of young adults (late teenagers and those in their early twenties) will develop infection with EBV. Symptoms and signs of infection will only appear in half of these and the reason for this is unknown

- The association of infectious mononucleosis and Hodgkin's lymphoma is strongest in young adults, but virus found in tumour cells is least frequently detected in tumours in this population
- It is still not clear whether primary infection with EBV in the form of infectious mononucleosis is a risk factor for EBV-positive Hodgkin's lymphoma
- It is possible that vaccination against EBV may modulate the course of infection and may reduce the risk of Hodgkin's lymphoma. This remains unproven
- Patients who fail to respond to chemotherapy or who relapse quickly after treatment may be cured with high-dose therapy and autologous stem cell transplantation

Further reading

Berthe MP, Aleman MD & Raemaekers JMM, et al. Involved-field radiotherapy for advanced Hodgkin's lymphoma. *New England Journal of Medicine* 2003; **348**: 2396–2406.

Diehl V, Franklin J & Pfreundschuh M, et al. Standard and increased-dose BEACOPP chemotherapy compared with COPP-ABVD for advanced Hodgkin's disease. *New England Journal of Medicine* 2003; **348**: 2386–2395.

Diehl V, Re D & Josting A. Hodgkin's disease: clinical manifestations, staging, and therapy. In: Hoffman R, Benz EK Jr, Shattil SK, Furie B, Cohen HJ, Silberstein LE, et al. eds. *Hematology: Basic Principles and Practice*, 4th edn. Churchill Livingstone, 2004: 1347–1377.

Hasenclever D & Diehl V. A prognostic score for advanced Hodgkin's disease. *New England Journal of Medicine* 1998; **339**: 1506.

Horning SJ. Risk, cure and complications in advanced Hodgkin lymphoma. asheducationbook.hematologylibrary.org/cgi/content/full/2007/1/197

Case 15 — A 53-year-old woman with discomfort under her left arm

Asia Khalid is a 53-year-old Pakistani woman who works as a part-time secretary. Over the last 3 weeks she has felt a discomfort under her left arm (axilla), when she was washing herself. In addition to her work, Asia regularly babysits for her two small grandchildren. She now finds it more tiring. Fifteen years earlier Asia had breast cancer in her right breast. She says that it was a small tumour and that she was treated with radical mastectomy (surgical removal of her breast and associated lymph nodes) and radiotherapy. She has been well since. She used to smoke but stopped when the breast cancer was discovered.

What is your differential diagnosis?

The discomfort (Asia has never used the word pain) is presumably associated with the local feeling of 'enlargement'. This could be caused by the following:

1 A cyst
2 Enlarged lymph nodes resulting from a malignancy of the lymphoid system, or
3 Metastases from a cancer, possibly a recurrence of her original disease

What should you concentrate on when taking the history?

Ask specific questions and link them to an event in Asia's personal life or a well-known public event. Had the swelling ever been painful and was it increasing in size? Was the swelling tender? Did she notice weight loss, fever or night sweats.

Asia said that the swelling was not painful but probably increased in size recently. Her weight was stable and there was no history of night sweats.

Haematology: Clinical Cases Uncovered. By S. McCann, R. Foà, O. Smith and E. Conneally. Published 2009 by Blackwell Publishing, ISBN: 978-1-4051-8322-2

What should be done next?

A full physical examination.

Asia appeared healthy and the only abnormal physical finding was a nodal mass in the left axilla.

What investigations should be carried out next?

A full blood count (Table 44) blood film (Fig. 100), biochemical screen and viral screen, a chest radiograph, a mammogram (radiological examination of the breast to detect cancers that cannot be felt clinically) and an ultrasound examination of the left axilla and the abdomen.

The blood film showed an increased number of 'atypical' cleaved lymphocytes (Fig. 100).

What would you tell the patient?

It is possible that it is a recurrence of her breast cancer (this is, understandably, her primary worry); however, the lymphocytosis suggests a blood disorder, therefore a lymph node biopsy is indicated. There is in no immediate danger, but further investigation is needed. Asia should continue with her normal daily activities. She should be reviewed as soon as the results of the tests become available.

Epstein–Barr virus (EBV) serology was negative and the biochemical screening showed a moderate increase in lactic dehydrogenase (LDH) to 605 IU/L (normal 230–450 IU/L), the other values being normal.
The mammography, chest radiograph and ultrasound of the abdomen were negative. The ultrasound examination of the left axilla confirmed the enlarged lymph node.

What now is your differential diagnosis?

Having excluded other possibilities (breast cancer recurrence, viral infections), an enlarged axillary lymph node,

Table 44 Results of the blood count.

	Patient's results	Normal range (female)
Hb	13.9 g/dL	11.5–16.4 g/dL
WBC	8.9 × 10⁹/L	4.0–11.0 × 10⁹/L (10³/μL)
Lymphocytes	6.0 × 10⁹/L	1.5–3.5 × 10⁹/L (10³/μL)
Neutrophils	2.9 × 10⁹/L	2.0–7.5 × 10⁹/L (10³/μL)
Platelets	210 × 10⁹/L	140–450 × 10⁹/L (10³/μL)

Hb, haemoglobin; WBC, white blood cell count.

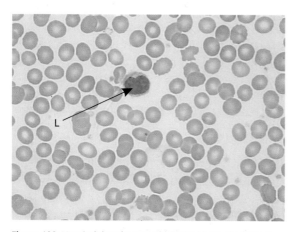

Figure 100 'Atypical' lymphoctytes (L) in the blood of a patient with infectious mononucleosis.

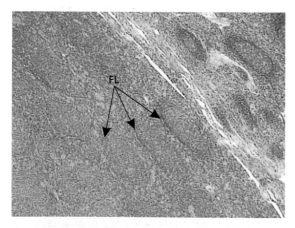

Figure 101 Lymph node with a follicular lymphoma (FL).

coupled to an increase in LDH, and the presence of nodal mass, fatigue and fever, strongly suggests the presence of an underlying lymphoma. Only a biopsy can provide a precise diagnosis.

KEY POINT

LDH is a ubiquitous enzyme found in all nucleated cells. It is found in the blood when cells die. This can be as a result of cancer, infarction of any tissue, premature destruction of red blood cells (haemolysis) or ineffective erythropoiesis (vitamin B_{12} or folate deficiency). It is a prominent finding in non-Hodgkin's lymphoma (NHL) and the degree of elevation of the LDH is indicative of the 'aggressiveness' of the lymphoma as it reflects cell death.

Why does the patient have a slight increase in lymphocytes (lymphocytosis), with other haematological values within the normal range?

If the diagnosis of a lymphoma is confirmed, the slight lymphocytosis could be caused by the presence of lymphoma cells in the blood. This requires further investigation.

How should the patient be managed?

Arrange to see the patient and her husband to explain that Asia needs to undergo an excision lymph node biopsy as soon as possible in order to make a diagnosis. This can be performed as an outpatient under local anaesthesia. She should continue with her various activities and the biopsy will be arranged with the surgeon within the week.

The procedure takes place 4 days later and the biopsy is sent unfixed to the pathologist. The conclusions of the histological examination are that the patient has NHL of follicular origin (Fig. 101).

What should the patient be told?

The lymph node biopsy has confirmed that she has non Hodgkin lymphoma (NHL). It should be explained that this is a malignancy of the lymphoid tissues that most often affects lymph nodes, that there are different forms of NHL and that she does not have any of the more aggressive forms. Asia's disease can be treated successfully and she should be referred to a haematologist as soon as possible.

What should be done next?

The physical findings were confirmed and nothing further emerged from the personal and family history.

The pathological evaluation of the lymph node confirmed that Asia had a follicular NHL. The pathological cells were of B-cell origin and were 'clonal' as they showed an immunoglobulin (Ig) κ light chain restriction.

NHL are a group of diseases that provide us with an insight into the mechanisms of malignancy. Lymph nodes are removed (excision biopsy means removing the complete node, instead of a piece of the node) for pathological examination and the cells made into a suspension and analysed by flow cytometry (Part 1). The node may also be cut into thin sections and immunological investigations carried out to demonstrate the 'clonality' (i.e. that the malignant cells are derived from a single cell) of the malignant cells.

Lymphomas are derived from B or T cells (the majority are derived from B cells). To demonstrate clonality, a functional test has been developed. B cells normally produce Ig. In a reactive or inflammatory (non-malignant) node, B cells produce Ig of different light chain types. In a malignant node, the Ig will be of a single light chain type, κ or λ (light chain restriction), indicating its origin from a single cell.

Another finding of great importance is that commonly there is transfer of genetic material from one chromosome to another in the malignant cells. Chromosomal material from chromosome 14 is translocated to chromosome 18, resulting in a resistance to apoptosis (programmed cell death) in the malignant cells. This gives us a clue to the mechanisms involved in the malignant cell and opens up new possibilities for treatment. These translocations and clonality in lymphoma cells can be demonstrated by flow cytometry, immunocytochemistry and genetic analysis.

Based on the diagnosis made, how could the increased number of lymphocytes in the patient's blood be more precisely investigated?

Flow cytometry (Part 1). Because the neoplastic cells are B cells with an Ig κ chain restriction, these cells can be easily looked for in the blood through a simple flow cytometry evaluation.

It was found that the patient had lymphoma cells in her blood.

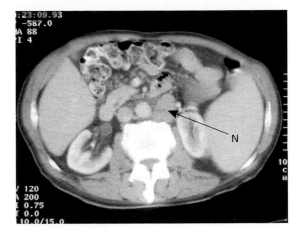

Figure 102 Computed tomography (CT) scan of the thorax was negative, while the CT of the abdomen showed enlarged lymph nodes (N).

What further investigations should be carried out?

A computed tomography (CT) scan of the abdomen and thorax and a bone marrow biopsy will help to evaluate the extent of disease.

The CT of the thorax was negative, while the CT of the abdomen showed enlarged lymph nodes (Fig. 102). The bone marrow biopsy showed a small infiltration of Ig κ lymphoma cells.

What are the practical implications of all these investigations?

To subdivide NHL into 'indolent' (slow growing) or 'aggressive' (rapidly growing) forms as these bear important prognostic implications. Patients with follicular lymphomas most often fall within the indolent subtype and less frequently under the aggressive subtype.

KEY POINT

Although the incidence is increasing the aetiology of most lymphomas is unknown. However, a number of lymphomas occur where a viral aetiology has been demonstrated. Denis Burkitt was the first to demonstrate the viral cause of a particular lymphoma in Africa. This was a lymphoma found in the jaw of children and was subsequently shown to be caused by EBV infection. However, EBV is not a cause of the common B or T cell lymphomas found in adults. EBV has been implicated in the lymphomas found in HIV infected patients and may have a role in some patients with Hodgkin's lymphoma.

What is the general approach to the management of patients with follicular lymphoma (NHL)?

The choice of treatment depends on the stage of the disease and the age and general health of the patient. Radiotherapy alone can be utilized for patients in the initial stages of the disease. Chemotherapy is usually utilized for patients with more advanced disease.

More recently, the combination of chemotherapy and the monoclonal antibody rituximab (induces apoptosis in malignant B cells via the CD20 antigen) has been successfully utilized.

Can you now construct an algorithm for the investigation of a patient with a large lymph node?

Yes.

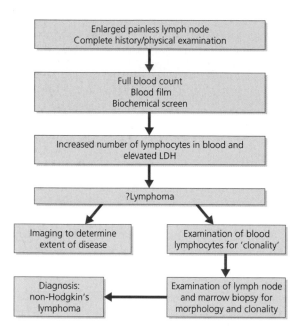

Outcome. Asia was treated with combination chemotherapy, after which she had a complete disappearance of symptoms and clinical and laboratory signs. However, monitoring of her disease indicated persistence of malignant B cells in her bone marrow after completing the chemotherapy programme. Asia was then given the anti-CD20 antibody, which induced a complete remission of her disease. Asia returned to 100% fitness, to work and enjoyed looking after her grandchildren again.

CASE REVIEW

A middle-aged women presents with a history of discomfort in her left axilla. She also complains of fatigue. The most important thing in the history is that she had breast cancer, which was treated 15 years earlier. It is extremely important when taking a history to enquire specifically about illness such as cancer, as it may have a major impact on the presenting complaint. It is probable that the original diagnosis she was given is correct, but it is possible that other tumours such as NHL could occur outside the lymph nodes and present as a primary breast mass. This would have implications for her current presentation. The finding of a fixed mass in the left axilla, with a previous history, makes one extremely suspicious of a recurrence of breast cancer. Breast cancer can recur as long as 20 years after the primary treatment. Breast cancer can occur in the second breast. The elevated LDH suggest cell death and this could be caused by recurrence of her breast cancer or other malignancy.

As is common in haemalogical diseases, careful examination of the blood film in this case proved to be extremely helpful. A marginal increase in the lymphocyte count together with abnormal appearing cells was a clue to the underlying diagnosis. Excision biopsy and examination by an experienced pathologist confirmed a diagnosis of NHL. It is extremely important to diagnose correctly in order to select appropriate therapy. Diagnostic techniques using immunocytochemistry or flow cytometry are extremely helpful in confirming the specific type of NHL, as in this case. Management of NHL virtually always includes combination chemotherapy with or without the addition of other agents such as monoclonal antibodies.

KEY POINTS

- Follicular lymphoma accounts for about one-third of NHL cases seen in adults
- The extent of the disease can be confirmed by examination of the peripheral blood and the bone marrow, radiography, CT scanning and positron emission tomography CT scanning (PET-CT). The uptake of the radiotracer ^{18}F-fluorodeoxyglucose is indicative of active tumour metabolism. This test is used to establish

Continued

if the patient has achieved a complete remission following appropriate therapies

- In spite of current therapy, most patients will experience a relapse of their original disease over time but remissions may last for years
- A significant number of these patients can be cured with further high-dose combination chemotherapy followed by autologous stem cell transplantation. Allogeneic stem cell transplantation may be an option in younger patients
- The presumed cells of origin for follicular lymphoma are germinal centre B cells. These cells express BCL2 and BCL6 proteins
- Virtually all cases of follicular lymphoma express t(14;18) involving rearrangement of the *BCL2* gene. The rearranged gene is constitutively active and produces a protein that blocks apoptosis
- The BCL2 protein is not detected in normal resting B cells
- Gene expression profiling may be able to detect 'survival associated signature' genes

Further reading

Kipps TJ. Advances in classification and therapy of indolent B-cell malignancies. *Seminars in Oncology* 2002; **29** (Suppl 2): 98 104.

Rambaldi A, Lazzari M, Manzoni C, *et al*. Monitoring of minimal residual disease after CHOP and rituximab in previously untreated patients with follicular lymphoma. *Blood* 2002; **99**: 856–862.

Reiser M & Diehl V. Current treatment of follicular non-Hodgkin's lymphoma. *European Journal of Cancer* 2002; **38**: 1167–1172.

Salles GA, Natkunam Y & Moloney DG. Follicular lymphoma. asheducationbook.hematologylibrary.org/cgi/content/full/2007/ Accessed in 2007.

Schiller GJ. ed. *Chronic Leukemias and Lymphomas: Biology, Pathophysiology and Clinical Management*. Humana Press, 2003.

Staudt LM. Molecular diagnosis of the hematologic cancers. *New England Journal of Medicine* 2003; **348**: 1777–1785.

Case 16 A 65-year-old red-faced man with a 'smoker's cough'

Richard Spring, a 65-year-old man, was encouraged to go to his family doctor by his wife. She thought his cough was getting worse and he seemed a little confused lately. He retired 1 year ago from a clerical job in an insurance company. For the last 6 months Richard felt a little 'muzziness' and said that the crossword, which he had completed every day for the last 30 years, was now becoming difficult. Some days he did not even bother read the newspaper. He had been a cigarette smoker all his adult life and he thought his chronic cough, worse in winter, had deteriorated recently.

What is your differential diagnosis?

Chronic bronchitis and/or emphysema are likely because he has smoked cigarettes all of his adult life and has a chronic cough. A change in the pattern of a 'smoker's cough', hoarseness or coughing blood (haemoptysis) are highly suspicious of lung cancer. Lung cancer can spread (metastasize) to the brain and produce symptoms of poor concentration or 'muzziness'.

A pulmonary embolus, associated or not with cancer, and secondary infection.

A viral pneumonia, which is often followed by secondary bacterial pneumonia in elderly people.

How would you approach this patient?

Take a full history with particular reference to hoarseness, haemoptysis, weight loss and precisely what the patient's wife meant by a change in the pattern of his cough. Ask about a history of high blood pressure or respiratory tract infections and a family history of cancer.

Haematology: Clinical Cases Uncovered. By S. McCann, R. Foà, O. Smith and E. Conneally. Published 2009 by Blackwell Publishing, ISBN: 978-1-4051-8322-2

Richard had about one respiratory tract infection yearly requiring antibiotics. He denied any change in his voice, haemoptysis, weight loss or a real change in the pattern of his cough. His cough did not keep him awake at night and he was trying to stop smoking.

Richard had two children, a son aged 40 and a daughter aged 42, both of whom were alive and well.

What should be done next?

A complete physical examination, including the cranial nerves and central nervous system. Measure the blood pressure; examine the urine and optic fundi.

There was no papilloedema (presence indicates raised intracranial pressure which could indicate a primary brain tumour or metastasis). He looked plethoric (Fig. 103). His blood pressure was elevated at 160/100 mm/Hg. The cranial nerves and central nervous system were intact. A few crackles were audible in both lung bases. The only other abnormality was an enlarged spleen, palpable 4 cm below the left costal margin in quiet inspiration (Figs 104 and 105). There was no blood or protein in the urine.

What else might you ask in view of his physical appearance?

Ask Richard and his wife if they had noticed a change in the patient's physical appearance in the last year, especially if his face was more 'purple–red' than it used to be.

Ask him if he has a photograph of himself a few years ago.

What investigations should be carried out?

A chest radiograph and ultrasound examination of the abdomen. A full blood count (Table 45), blood film and a biochemical screen.

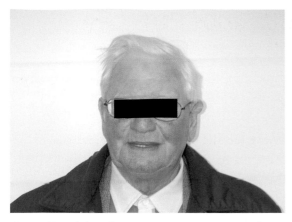

Figure 103 A plethoric face.

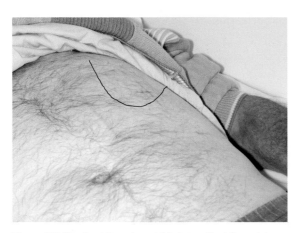

Figure 104 The tip of the spleen visible below the left coastal margin.

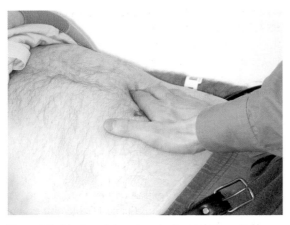

Figure 105 Palpation of the enlarged spleen.

Table 45 Results of the full blood count.

	Patient's results	Normal range
Hb	19.5 g/dL	13.5–17.5 g/dL
MCV	70.0 fL	76–96 fL (μm^3)
RBC	7.0×10^{12}/L	4.5–6.5×10^{12}/L (10^6/μL)
WBC	13.5×10^9/L	4.0–11.0×10^9/L (10^3/μL)
Platelets	625×10^9/L	150–450×10^9/L (10^3/μL)

Hb, haemoglobin; MCV, mean corpuscular volume; RBC, red cell count; WBC, white blood cell count.

> **KEY POINT**
>
> He should stop smoking immediately (nicotine substitutes or other supportive measures are frequently required). If patients stop smoking at 65 years and live for another 10 years they will significantly reduce the risk of developing lung cancer.

How should the patient be managed?

Richard should return in a few days for a further blood pressure measurement and the results of the blood tests.

The radiograph showed some hyperinflation of the chest, a normal heart size and no evidence of lung cancer.

Always request a lateral chest radiograph as this may reveal abnormalities not detected on a postero-anterior view which are obscured by the cardiac shadow.

The ultrasound examination confirmed an enlarged spleen. His blood pressure remained elevated at 150/100 mmHg.
Occasional large platelets were noted on the blood film. There was an elevated uric acid level 520 μmol/L (normal 150–470 μmol/L or 3.0–8.0 mg/dl.)

Now what is your differential diagnosis?

The haemoglobin and red cell count are both increased so the patient has erythrocytosis. The platelet count is also elevated so there could be a bone marrow problem causing an excess production of red cells and platelets. The patient also has a large spleen suggesting that there is some fundamental disturbance of the haematological system. The elevated uric acid could have been present for a long time and may reflect idiopathic hyperuricaemia or increased cell turnover.

How can you connect all the information?

Lung cancer could cause his cough and his 'muzziness' because of metastases in his brain. It is unusual to have a large spleen with metastatic cancer. The erythrocytosis could be secondary to chronic lung disease and hypoxia as a result of his cigarette smoking.

Some lung cancers secrete a hormone with 'erythropoietin-like' activity causing the raised red cell count. A raised platelet count can occur with any malignancy.

Other possibilities include diseases that cause a reduction in blood oxygen levels (hypoxaemia) such as a right to left shunt in the heart, heavy cigar smoking, chronic obstructive airways disease or a congenital high-affinity haemoglobin. A renal cyst producing 'erythropoietin-like' hormones. Polycythaemia vera (PV), a disease where there is overproduction of red cells (and sometimes white cells and platelets) in the bone marrow, should also be considered.

KEY POINT

Red cell production is a precisely regulated phenomenon (Fig. 106).

What should be done next?

He should be referred to hospital immediately for further investigations.

Richard was given an appointment for the following week to see a haematologist.

What would the haematologist do?

Repeat the history and physical examination, which confirmed the plethoric appearance, enlarged spleen and elevated blood pressure.

What further investigations should be carried out?

Sputum examination for malignant cells, which, if present, would indicate lung cancer.

The chest radiograph findings were confirmed. Pulse oxymetry was carried out (Fig. 107). This revealed an oxygen saturation of 97% (normal 96–100%).

How reliable is pulse oxymetry in detecting hypoxaemia in the patient?

Very reliable. Thus, hypoxaemia is not the reason for the increased red cell count. Arterial blood gases should be measured if the oxymetry is abnormal and the patient investigated to elucidate the cause.

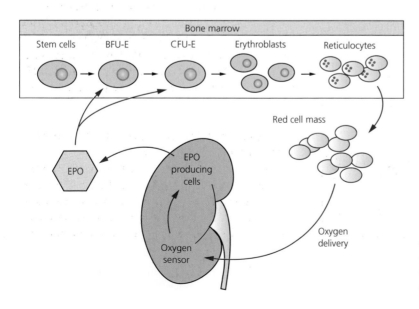

Figure 106 Interactions between erythropoietin (EPO), the kidney and oxygenation. BFU-E, burst-forming unit erythroid; CFU-E, colony-forming unit erythroid.

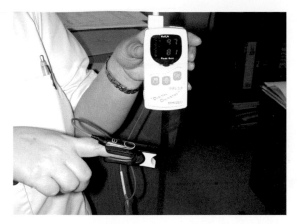

Figure 107 Pulse oxymetry.

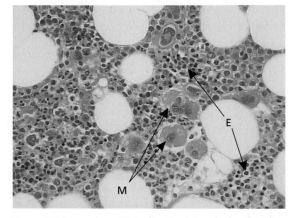

Figure 109 Bone marrow biopsy showing red cell hyperplasia. E, erythroid precursors; M, megakaryocytes.

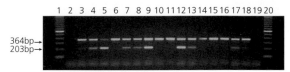

Figure 108 Identification of the *JAK2* V617F mutation in patients with myeloproliferative disorders including polycythaemia vera (PV). Lanes 1 and 20, contain a DNA ladder; lanes 2 and 19, polymerase chain reaction (PCR) negative controls; lanes 3 and 18, PCR-positive controls; lanes 4–9, PV patients; lanes 10–13, essential thrombocythaemia (ET) patients; lanes 14–17, primary myelofibrosis (PMF) patients.

Table 46 Results of erythropoietin levels.

	Patient's results	Normal range
Erythopoietin	8.5 IU/mL	6.0–25.0 IU/mL

KEY POINT

The most common cause of hypoxaemia is chronic obstructive airways disease secondary to chronic cigarette smoking.

What would the haematologist do?

Measure the level of erythropoietin (EPO) in the plasma and send blood for analysis of a *JAK2* kinase mutation. See Table 46.

How can these results be interpreted?

The EPO level is normal. This excludes a secondary cause for the erythrocytosis, i.e. a hypoxaemic drive to produce more EPO. The mutant kinase, identified as the V617F mutation is virtually diagnostic of PV as it is found in >95% of cases.

The *JAK2* kinase analysis is carried out using a technique known as allele-specific polymerase chain reaction (PCR). The extra band represents the mutant kinase (Fig. 108). DNA is extracted from whole blood and is subjected to an allele-specific PCR which identifies a control band (364 bp) in all patient samples and a smaller band (203 bp) in those patients in whom the *JAK2* V617F is present.

How useful is the measurement of EPO in making a diagnosis?

It is sometimes useful. If there is a hypoxaemic state the levels of EPO are elevated reflecting the increased drive to produce red cells. However, if a tumour or a renal cyst is secreting EPO, the serum levels are not elevated and samples from the blood vessel draining the tumour or directly from the renal cyst are taken. In PV the serum levels of erythropoietin are usually normal or decreased.

What do the results so far indicate?

The patient has an overactive bone marrow for a reason other than hypoxia. The clinical and laboratory findings strongly support a diagnosis of PV.

What other investigations would the haematologist perform at this stage?

A bone marrow biopsy (Fig. 109).

Since the discovery of the *JAK2* kinase mutation the requirement to carry out a bone marrow examination has become very controversial. The bone marrow findings in Richard's case support a diagnosis of PV but are not diagnostic.

PV is a disease usually seen in people over the age of 60 years. It is caused by a clonal expansion (derived from a single clone of bone marrow stem cells) in the marrow leading to excess production of red blood cells, granulocytes and platelets. The *JAK2* kinase mutation is acquired (not congenital) and the result is a change in the function of the EPO receptor and an uninterrupted proliferation of marrow cells. Like other clonal disorders of the marrow there may be chromosomal abnormalities. Deletions (partial loss) of chromosome 20 are the most common findings.

What clinical problems would he experience if untreated?

Vascular problems in the arterial and venous circulation. The increased number of circulating red cells and red cell mass will increase the blood viscosity. The increased platelet numbers, cigarette smoking and high blood pressure will also increase the risk of arterial vascular problems.

Can you now construct an algorithm to investigate a patient with erythrocytosis?

Yes.

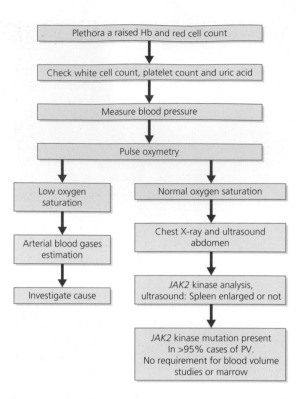

Outcome. A diagnosis of PV was made. Richard's blood pressure was treated and he was given oral chemotherapy with hydroxyurea until his platelet count returned to normal (150–$450 \times 10^9/L$ or $10^3/\mu L$). He was venesected at weekly intervals until his haemoglobin returned to normal (13.5–17.5 g/dL) and encouraged to stop smoking. Richard's symptoms disappeared and he returned to his daily crossword puzzles.

KEY POINT

Avoid the use of diuretics when treating high blood pressure in patients with PV. Diuretics decrease the plasma volume, therefore increasing the haematocrit and risk of vascular events. Remember, do not venesect a patient if the platelet count is elevated. The platelet count will rise further following venesection and could cause a 'stroke'.

CASE REVIEW

An elderly man is plethoric and confused. The diagnosis could be lung cancer in view of his smoking history and it is important to rule this out as the prognosis for most patients is extremely poor with a survival measured in months. The important clue in this man's case is the preliminary blood findings. The combination of an elevated haemoglobin or haematocrit together with a low MCV is indicative of PV. The low MCV in this case indicates reduced iron stores, which could be caused by the rapid red cell turnover or the possibility of concomitant gastrointestinal tract bleeding. Other causes of erythrocytosis such as hypoxaemia should have a normal MCV and if the MCV is decreased the haemoglobin and/or haematocrit will also be reduced.

The most important investigation in a patient with erythrocytosis is to find out if the patient is hypoxaemic or not. Hypoxaemia will open a number of possibilities, the most common of which is chronic obstructive airway disease. Any cause of right to left shunting will result in the presence of deoxygenated blood in the systemic circulation. Congenital heart disease or arteriovenous malformations may lead to erythrocytosis but the former is usually diagnosed in childhood.

Rare causes of erythrocytosis without hypoxaemia and excluding PV are tumours secreting EPO (renal, cerebellar, ovarian and others). Congenital high-affinity haemoglobins will behave similarly and are extremely rare. Their oxygenation dissociation curve is different to normal adult haemoglobin (Hb A).

In this case the suspicion of PV because of the clinical, haematological and laboratory findings was confirmed by the molecular test. The presence of the JAK2 mutation has revolutionized the diagnosis of PV and to a lesser extent the other myeloproliferative diseases such as essential thrombocythaemia (ET) and primary myelofibrosis (PMF). The need to measure red cell mass and blood volumes is almost redundant and new criteria for the diagnosis of PV are currently being discussed.

KEY POINTS

- For many years the fundamental defect in PV was believed to be an uncontrolled proliferation of erythrocytes and to a lesser extent neutrophils and platelets. Other clinical states were recognized which were probably related to PV but the clinical manifestations were different. These disorders include ET and PMF, which are characterized by a high platelet count and marrow fibrosis, respectively
- These disorders have been unified within a concept of so-called 'myeloproliferative diseases' for many years and it is only within the past few years that an acquired mutation in a kinase has been found in all three diseases
- The JAK family of intracellular kinases activate downstream proteins involved in signal transduction and are therefore very important in cell proliferation. Normally, the EPO receptor undergoes a conformational change after ligand binding (EPO to the EPO receptor). This causes a conformational change in JAK and leads to activation of other transcription factors and regulation of selected genes in the nucleus
- The JAK2 V617F mutant binds to the cytoplasmic domain of intracellular and cell-surface EPO receptor and promotes ligand-independent signalling
- It is believed that interaction between mutated JAK2 and the EPO receptor contributes to the pathobiology of PV and ET by causing uncontrolled cell proliferation
- The V617F mutation is found in 95% of patients with PV, 50% with ET and 50% of PMF patients
- This molecular defect is similar to that found in chronic myeloid leukaemia and a number of drugs that specifically inhibit the mutated kinase are currently under investigation (Case 10)

Further reading

Hoffbrand AV, Moss PAH & Pettit JE. *Essential Haematology*, 5th edn. Blackwell Science, 2006: 230–240.

Means RT Jr. Polycythemia vera. In: Lee GR, Foerster J, Lukene J, Paraskevas F, Greer J & Rodgers G, eds. *Wintrobe's Clinical Hematology*, Vol 2, 10th edn. Williams and Wilkins, 1999: 2374–2389.

Skoda R. The genetic basis of myeloproliferative disorders. asheducationbook.hematologylibrary.org/cgi/content/full/2007/1/1 Accessed in 2007.

Tefferi A. *Classification, diagnosis and management of myeloproliferative diseases in the JAK2V67F era.* asheducationbook. haematologylibrary.org/2006.

Case 17 A 28-year-old woman who suddenly started bruising

Mary Welles, a 28-year-old web designer, went to her doctor because she had noticed bruising on her arms and legs for 3–4 days. The bruises were not painful but were increasing in number every day.

What is your differential diagnosis?

Spontaneous bruising could be caused by a decreased platelet count (thrombocytopenia), abnormal platelet function or inflammation of blood vessels resulting in leakage of red cells into the skin (vasculitis). In this age group a low platelet count would be the most likely possibility. Thrombocytopenia can be caused by bone marrow failure resulting from aplasia, invasion of the bone marrow by cancer, leukaemia, deficiency of vitamin B_{12} or folate, or anything causing a shortened platelet lifespan such as immune destruction or sequestration in an enlarged spleen.

What should be done?

A full history, with particular emphasis on recent (viral) infection and medications.

Mary had no fever or other evidence of infection and did not admit to taking any medications. Many medications are associated with thrombocytopenia although it is usually a rare occurrence (Table 47). Heavy alcohol ingestion can impair platelet production.

What should be done next?

A physical examination.

The examination revealed that Mary was a healthy looking young woman with bruising and petechiae on her arms and legs (Fig. 110). There was no other abnormality; specifically,

the spleen was not palpable and lymph nodes were not enlarged. There was no evidence of IV drug ingestion.

How should the patient be managed?

A full blood count (Table 48), blood film (Fig. 111), coagulation and biochemical screen should be carried out immediately. Mary should be requested to return later that afternoon for the results.

The coagulation screen was normal and the blood film confirmed a reduced platelet count (Fig. 111).

How do you interpret the full blood count and coagulation screen?

The platelet count is obviously extremely low. This would probably explain the spontaneous bruising. The haemoglobin and white cell count are normal, making bone marrow failure an unlikely diagnosis. The absence of abnormal physical signs such as a large spleen or lymphadenopathy make the diagnosis of cancer or a haematological malignancy unlikely.

> **KEY POINT**
>
> The coagulation screen is not influenced by the platelet count as a platelet substitute is added to the test material. Therefore, thrombocytopenia does not cause a prolonged prothrombin time (PT) or activated partial thromboplastin time (APTT).

What should be done next?

Mary should be referred to a specialist immediately.

What advice should be given to the patient?

Mary should be advised not to take aspirin or any anti-inflammatory drugs. She should rest that evening and see the specialist the following day.

Haematology: Clinical Cases Uncovered. By S. McCann, R. Foà, O. Smith and E. Conneally. Published 2009 by Blackwell Publishing, ISBN: 978-1-4051-8322-2

Table 47 Some of the drugs that have been associated with thrombocytopenia. This list is not comprehensive and does not include chemotherapeutic agents that cause myelosuppression.

Quinine, heparin, gold salts, antimicrobials (e.g. cephalosporins, ciprofloxacin, clarithromycin, fluconazole, fusidic acid, gentamicin, nilidixic acid, penicillins, pentamidine, rifampicin, sulfamethoxazole, vancomycin) non-steroidal anti-inflammatory drugs (NSAIDs)

Cardiac medications and diuretics (e.g. digoxin, amiodarone, procainamide, captopril, diazoxide, alpha-methyldopa, acetazolamide, chlorothiazide, chlortalidone, furosemide, hydrochlorothiazide, spironolactone, benzodiazepines)

Anti-epileptic drugs, H2-antagonists, glibenclamide, retinoids, antihistamines

Antidepressants

Table 48 Results of full blood count.

	Patient's results	Normal range
Hb	12.0 g/dL	11.5–16.4 g/dL
WBC	5×10^9/L	$4.0–11.0 \times 10^9$/L (10^3/µL)
Neutrophils	3.5×10^9/L	$2.0–7.5 \times 10^9$/L (10^3/µL)
Lymphocytes	1.5×10^9/L	$1.5–3.5 \times 10^9$/L (10^3/µL)
Platelets	15×10^9/L	$140–450 \times 10^9$/L (10^3/µL)

Hb, haemoglobin; WBC, white blood cell count.

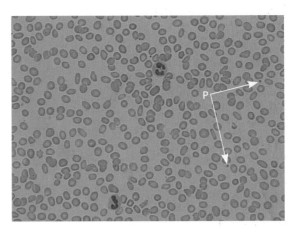

Figure 111 Blood film showing few platelets (P). In a normal individual, 10–25 platelets are expected in a field of this magnification.

❘ *The next day a haematologist reviewed her.*

What would the haematologist do?
Repeat the physical examination, the blood count and look at the blood film (Fig. 111).

> **KEY POINT**
>
> Remember to include examination of the retina. Bleeding into the retina can cause blindness if it occurs in the area of the macula, but also can be a 'window' to look at small blood vessels and predict the possibility of an intracranial bleed.

The blood counts were unchanged (Table 48) and the blood film (Fig. 111) confirmed a low platelet count. There were no abnormal white cells present, making the diagnosis of leukaemia unlikely.

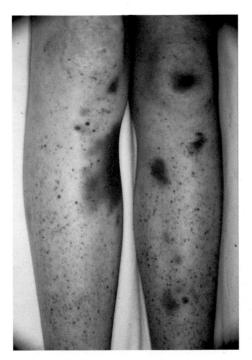

Figure 110 Extensive bruising and petechiae.

> **KEY POINT**
>
> Aspirin or anti-inflammatory drugs diminish platelet function by inhibition of cyclo-oxygenase. The inhibition induced by aspirin is irreversible and platelet function will only recover following synthesis and release of new platelets from the bone marrow.

What further tests should the haematologist carry out?

A biochemical screen and an ultrasound of the abdomen.

The biochemical screen was normal and the abdominal ultrasound revealed a normal spleen size with no intra-abdominal masses or lymphadenopathy.

What other serological investigation should be carried out?

A screening test for HIV infection.

What precautions should be taken before carrying out this test?

The patient should be informed of the possible diagnosis in view of the test being positive. A full history of possible exposure to HIV and patient consent should be obtained.

Now what is your differential diagnosis?

The probability now is that of immune platelet destruction. The absence of physical signs other than purpura, and the normal haemoglobin and white cell count make the diagnosis of a haematological malignancy or cancer unlikely. Although Mary did not admit to ingestion of medications or recreational drugs these cannot be excluded by history alone. The outcome of the HIV test is awaited therefore a positive test is still a possibility.

KEY POINT

The absence of an admission of exposure to risky sexual activity or drug abuse is not adequate to rule this out as a possible diagnosis as many patients are afraid or embarrassed to give an accurate history.

How would you manage this patient?

Mary should be admitted to hospital and orders given that she should not receive any intramuscular injections (Fig. 112), aspirin or other non-steroidal anti-inflammatory drugs.

What would the haematologist do next?

Carry out a bone marrow aspirate and biopsy (Fig. 113).

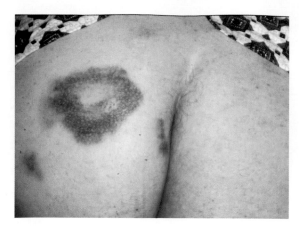

Figure 112 A large haematoma at an injection site in a patient with a low platelet count.

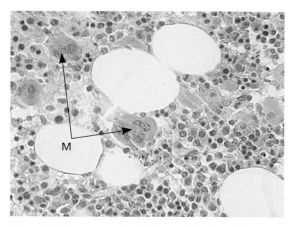

Figure 113 Bone marrow showing increased numbers of megakaryocytes (M).

The bone marrow aspirate and biopsy revealed an increased number of platelet precursors (megakaryocytes) and no abnormal cells.

How can you connect the appearance of the bone marrow with the low platelet count and the absence of a large spleen?

The increased numbers of megakaryocytes (platelet precursors) in the bone marrow suggests that platelet production is normal. The decreased number of platelets in the blood therefore suggests that there is premature destruction of platelets. Platelet numbers may be decreased in the presence of a large spleen as pooling may occur.

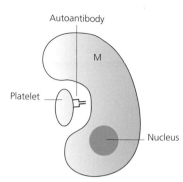

Figure 114 Macrophage (M) in the spleen engulfing an autoantibody and the platelet to which it is attached.

What diagnosis should be considered at this stage?

Autoimmune thrombocytopenic purpura (ITP). In ITP an autoantibody is formed, for reasons unknown, against a protein on the platelet membrane. The antibody adheres to the platelet membrane and is phagocytosed by macrophages in the reticuloendothelial system, primarily in the spleen. When engulfing the Fc receptor of the autoantibody, the macrophage also engulfs the platelet and the platelet is destroyed (Fig. 114). If the rate of destruction of platelets exceeds the compensatory increased production by the bone marrow (the marrow can increase the production by 6–7 times), the platelet count will fall and levels may drop to $<10 \times 10^9/L$ ($10^3/\mu L$).

What drugs in common use can be associated with a low platelet count?

Quinine, the antibiotics co-trimoxazole (Septrin) and rifampicin.

What drug commonly used in hospitals can cause a low platelet count?

Heparin. Heparin-induced thrombocytopenia–thrombosis syndrome (HITTS) may occur if patients are given heparin to prevent or treat venous thrombosis. The syndrome occurs because heparin induces platelet clumping leading to further thrombosis, both venous and arterial, and a low platelet count.

At what platelet level is there a danger of spontaneous intracranial bleeding?

It depends on the mechanism of the low platelet count. If the low platelet count is caused by premature destruc-

tion, the young platelets, which are released from the bone marrow, have excellent function and bleeding rarely occurs into the brain even if the platelet count is $<10 \times 10^9/L$ ($10^3/\mu L$).

However, if the low platelet count is caused by bone marrow failure, then a platelet count of $<10 \times 10^9/L$ ($10^3/\mu L$) may result in a high risk of intracranial bleeding.

How can the presence of a normal size spleen be reconciled with the diagnosis of ITP?

In a patient with ITP, as in Mary's case, the spleen is not enlarged. Although there is increased activity in the spleen the organ is always of normal size.

> **KEY POINT**
>
> The finding of an enlarged spleen in a patient with a low platelet count indicates a diagnosis other than ITP.

What syndrome may present with thrombocytopenia and an enlarged spleen?

Systemic lupus erythematosus (SLE). In this autoimmune disease, which is seen predominantly in young females, skin rashes, arthralgia and renal impairment are seen. The low platelet count is immune-mediated.

What diagnostic test result would exclude a diagnosis of SLE?

Absence of anti-DNA antibodies.

What are the principles of management of ITP?

In children, observation and conservative management is usually adequate (Table 49). In adults, if a low platelet count is accompanied by bleeding then treatment should be initiated in hospital using corticosteroids or intravenous immunoglobulins.

What are the potential hazards of giving immunoglobulin derived from human donor plasma?

There is always a risk of transmission of known or unknown viruses or other infectious agents, e.g. prions, when products derived from human plasma are used. The combination of intensive blood donor screening including a detailed medical history and measures taken

Table 49 Clinical course of autoimmune thrombocytopenic purpura (ITP) differs in children and adults.

Children	Adults
Usually of acute onset	Nearly always chronic
	Duration of >14 days
Commonly follows a viral infection	Rarely preceded by a viral infection
Nearly always self-limiting	
Treatment rarely required	Rarely recovers without treatment

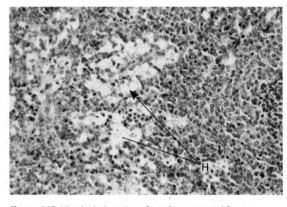

Figure 115 Histological section of a spleen removed from a patient with autoimmune thrombocytopenic purpura (ITP). H, histiocytes.

for inactivation of viruses reduces the risk substantially (Case 20).

In the event of failure of medical therapy and persistent thrombocytopenia and bleeding, what further interventions might be considered?
Splenectomy (Fig. 115).

How does removal of the spleen compromise the patient?
Individuals without a spleen are more *susceptible* to overwhelming infection with Gram-positive encapsulated bacteria (*Streptococcus pneumonia*, *Haemophilus influenza* and meningococcus).

What precautions should be taken prior to removal of the spleen?
Vaccination against the above.

What other precaution should be taken after the spleen is removed?
Administration of penicillin or erythromycin.

For how long should this treatment be administered after splenectomy?
For life.

Can you construct an algorithm to investigate a patient with purpura?
Yes.

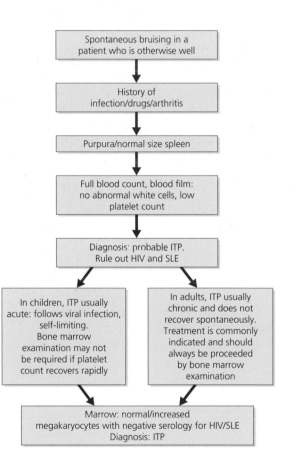

> **KEY POINT**
>
> The diagnosis of ITP is one of exclusion as there is no specific test for this condition.

CASE REVIEW

This young woman presented with what appeared to be spontaneous onset of bruising. The immediate fear for the patient and the doctor is that she has a serious haematological disorder such as acute leukaemia.

Two things should reassure the doctor. First, there are no other physical signs, although patients with acute leukaemia may present with bruising only. The second reassuring sign is the blood count. It would be extremely rare to have acute leukaemia with a normal haemoglobin and white blood cell count. Almost all cases of leukaemia in adults will have some degree of anaemia and an abnormal white cell count. Most of them will have some evidence of infection.

The diagnosis of ITP is by exclusion as there is no specific test. Although somewhat controversial in children, it is always advisable to carry out a bone marrow aspirate to exclude a more sinister diagnosis such as malignancy. Do not let a low platelet count inhibit you from carrying out a bone marrow examination.

In adults, ITP is usually chronic and may prove difficult to treat. It is important not to use large doses of corticosteroids for prolonged periods as this will cause severe toxicity. Failure to respond to steroids in a number of weeks requires an alternative approach to treatment.

> **KEY POINTS**
>
> - The amount of bleeding for a given platelet count is usually less if the aetiology is immune rather than induced by chemotherapy. This is probably because platelets are younger in situations where there is immune destruction and platelet function tends to be better when compared to thrombocytopenia induced by chemotherapy
> - Treatment for refractory ITP may be an indication for use of the monoclonal antibody anti-CD20 (rituximab). This may be useful in adults and children. Serum sickness and prolonged neutropenia have been reported and the drug should only be used by specialists and preferably within a prospective clinical trial
> - Recent evidence suggests that in some patients, platelet production may be suboptimal in the bone marrow and that this may contribute to the low platelet count

Further reading

Behtan P, Bussel J. Refractory immune thrombocytopenic purpurea: current strategies for investigation and management. *British Journal of Haematology* 2008; **143**(1): 16–26.

British Committee for Standards in Haematology General Haematology Task Force. Guidelines for the investigation and management of idiopathic thrombocytopenic purpura in adults, children and in pregnancy. *British Journal of Haematology* 2003; **120**: 574–596.

George JN, Raskob GE, Shar SR, *et al.* Drug induced thrombocytopenia: a systematic review of published case reports. *Annals of Internal Medicine* 2001; **129**: 886–890.

Hoffbrand AV, Moss PAH & Pettit JE. *Essential Haematology*, 5th edn. Blackwell Science, Oxford, 2006: 250–260.

Watson HG, Keeling DM; BCSH Taskforce in Haemostasis and Thrombosis. The management of heparin induced thrombocytopaenia. *British Journal of Haematology* 2006; **135**: 259–269.

Case 18 Delivery of a newborn baby boy that went wrong

Anne Percy was admitted to the delivery suite in her local maternity hospital. Because Anne failed to 'progress in labour' forceps were used to deliver the head of the baby. After delivery the midwife noticed that the baby had a large haematoma (blood under the skin) on the scalp.

What should the midwife do?

Call the neonatologist immediately.

What should the neonatologist do?

A full physical examination of the baby.

Physical examination was normal apart from the haematoma on the scalp (Fig. 116).

What is the differential diagnosis?

A congenital bleeding disorder should be suspected. Small haematomas may occur in the scalp after a difficult delivery especially if a ventouse vacuum is used but this haematoma was unexpectedly large for a forceps delivery. The most likely diagnosis is of a coagulation abnormality. Congenital factor VIII or IX deficiency would be the most likely diagnosis. Other coagulation deficiencies such as factor X, V or II are extremely rare as is an abnormal fibrinogen or fibrinogen deficiency. Factor VII deficiency occurs in specific ethnic groups. Rare severe forms of von Willebrand disease may present in this manner. A platelet deficiency would present with generalized purpura as well as a haematoma.

What should the neonatologist do next?

Reassure Anne and tell her that there appears to be a problem but the extent and nature is as yet ill-defined. The neonatologist should take a history from the mother.

Haematology: Clinical Cases Uncovered. By S. McCann, R. Foà, O. Smith and E. Conneally. Published 2009 by Blackwell Publishing, ISBN: 978-1-4051-8322-2

What questions should be asked to find out if Anne had a history of abnormal bleeding?

Did Anne ever have bleeding following dental extraction or surgery? Ask specifically about tonsillectomy as that is a severe haemostatic challenge and a negative history may be helpful. Did bleeding occur into joints or was easy bruising a feature? Did Anne play any contact sports as a child? Did anybody in her family have any of the above?

Anne's history was negative and she said that as far as she was aware there was no family history of abnormal bleeding.

> **KEY POINT**
>
> Coagulation factor deficiencies typically have abnormal bleeding into muscles and joints. Bleeding brought about by a platelet deficiency causes bleeding from mucosal surfaces and bruising. Excessive menstrual blood loss may be the only evidence of a bleeding disorder (e.g. von Willebrand disease).

How helpful is a patient's history when trying to assess menorrhagia (excessive menstrual blood loss)?

Frequently it is unhelpful. Each woman's definition of menorrhagia can be different.

> **KEY POINT**
>
> Menorrhagia is defined as greater than 80 mL on three consecutive periods and laboratory-based assays are the only way to measure it accurately. Unfortunately, these tests are unavailable and the diagnosis is commonly made by change in pattern of bleeding and iron deficiency anaemia without any other explanation.

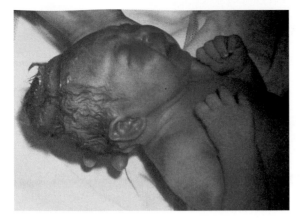

Figure 116 Haematoma on the scalp of a newborn.

Table 51 Results of the coagulation screen.

	Patient's result	Normal range (newborn)
Prothrombin time (PT)	14.2 s	10.1–15.9 secs
Activated partial thromboplastin time (APTT)	82.0 s	31.3–54.5 secs
Thrombin time (TT)	14.8 s	12.7–20.2 secs
Fibrinogen	2.90 g/L	1.67–3.99 g/L (150–360 mg/dL)

Table 50 Results of the blood count and coagulation screen.

	Patient's results	Normal range (newborn)
Hb	11.6 g/dL	14.9–23.7 g/dL
MCV	120 fL	100–125 fL (μm^3)
Platelets	440 × 10⁹/L	140–450 × 10⁹/L (10³/μL)

Hb, haemoglobin; MCV, mean corpuscular volume.

Table 52 Result of the reticulocyte count.

	Patient's result	Normal range (newborn)
Reticulocytes	134 × 10⁹/L	110–150 × 10⁹/L (0.5–1.5%)

Why is the family history of the mother important?

Because the bleeding occurred at the time of delivery it is possible that the child has a congenital bleeding disorder. As congenital bleeding disorders are commonly familial, a family history would be useful to confirm this possibility.

What should be done next?

A bleeding history should be taken from the mother. Ask if she has any brothers and if any of them have had abnormal bleeding. The common inherited coagulation disorders are due to an abnormality on the X chromosome therefore the father or his siblings will not have a bleeding history.

What tests should be performed to clarify the diagnosis?

A full blood count (Table 50), platelet count and coagulation screen (Table 51).

How can the full blood count be interpreted?

The baby is anaemic. This may reflect bleeding that has occurred into the baby's scalp. The platelet count is normal, excluding thrombocytopenia as a cause of the bleeding.

What further tests could be carried out to elucidate the cause of the baby's anaemia?

A reticulocyte count (Table 52).

How can this result be interpreted?

The reticulocyte count and MCV are normal for a newborn baby.

Now what is your differential diagnosis?

The activated partial thromboplastin time (APTT) is prolonged and the prothrombin time (PT) is normal. This indicates an abnormality of the 'intrinsic clotting system', which is measured by the APTT (Fig. 117). This is probably haemophilia because a deficiency of factor VIII or IX would result in a prolonged APTT with a normal PT

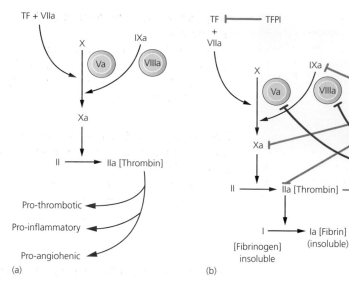

Figure 117 (a) Blood coagulation is initiated (initiation phase) when tissue factor (TF), expressed after injury to cell wall (e.g. endothelial, monocytic cells), is exposed to FVIIa in the bloodstream. TF–FVIIa complex in turn activates FIX to FIXa and FX to FXa. FIXa with its cofactor FVIIIa in turn also activates FX to FXa (amplification phase). FXa with its cofactor FVa activates prothrombin (II) to thrombin (IIa) (propagation phase). Thrombin converts soluble fibrinogen to insoluble fibrin. Thrombin is not only prothrombotic but activates platelets and is pro-inflammatory and promotes new vessel formation. (b) The initiation phase of coagulation is controlled by inhibiting the complex of TF, FVIIa and FXa by tissue factor pathway inhibitor (TFPI). The amplification phase of coagulation is blocked by the protein C pathway. Protein C (PC) is activated by a complex of thrombin, thrombomodulin (TM), and endothelial protein C receptor (EPCR) to activated protein C (APC) which in association with protein S (PS) inactivates FVa and FVIIa. The thrombin formed in the propagation phase is controlled by antithrombin (AT).

and also cause bleeding and would be the most common congenital coagulation disorder. Severe von Willebrand disease is still a possibility but very rare. Factor II or fibrinogen deficiency would result in a prolongation of both tests.

> **KEY POINT**
>
> The PT and APTT are not influenced by the platelet count as a substitute for platelets is added during the testing of a patient's plasma.

What other possibility could explain the abnormal coagulation screen in the baby?

Vitamin K deficiency results in impaired synthesis of factors II, VII, IX, X, protein C and S, and may cause haemorrhagic disease in newborn infants. This is unlikely here as the PT is normal and both the PT and APTT would be prolonged with vitamin K deficiency.

What should be done if vitamin K deficiency is suspected?

Vitamin K should be given intravenously.

> **KEY POINT**
>
> Vitamin K should not be given intramuscularly as the baby obviously has a bleeding defect and this could cause a haematoma (bleeding into a muscle).

What should the mother be told at this stage?

Anne should be told that it is likely that the baby has a congenital bleeding disorder. A specific diagnosis should be available within 24–48 hours. Most congenital bleeding disorders can be easily treated.

What further blood tests should be ordered?

Measurement of the factor VIII and IX level in the baby's blood.

Table 53 Results of factor VII and IX assays.

	Patient's result	Normal range
Factor VIII	0%	22–139%
Factor IX	64%	10–66%

Factor VIII and IX deficiency are the most common inherited bleeding disorders that present with bleeding in the neonatal period. Factor VIII deficiency is six times most common than factor IX deficiency. The results of factor VIII and IX assay are shown in Table 53.

What is the diagnosis?

Factor VIII is absent in the baby's plasma. This is compatible with a diagnosis of severe haemophilia A.

KEY POINT

Haemophilia is caused by mutations of the *FVIII* gene (haemophilia A) or *FIX* gene (haemophilia B) on the X chromosome. Approximately 1 male child in 5000 is affected by haemophilia A. Over 200 mutations in the large and complex *FVIII* gene lead to inadequate synthesis of FVIII and hence thrombin generation is impaired. Approximately 50% of all haemophilia A is caused by an inversion of intron 22, which simplifies the diagnosis and genetic counselling.

Why is the gender of the child important?

The gene for factor VIII is present on the X chromosome and this disease is therefore an 'X-linked disease'. This means that the disease manifests itself in boys but that girls can be 'carriers' (Figure 118).

How often is a family history of bleeding obtained in children with haemophilia?

About 30–50% of children with haemophilia have no family history of abnormal bleeding. This is because of spontaneous mutations in the factor VIII or IX gene.

What level of factor VIII is present in carriers (girls who pass on haemophilia to their children)?

The levels of factor VIII in carriers are variable because of random X chromosome inactivation known as 'lyonization' (Fig. 119).

As a diagnosis of haemophilia A has now been made what advice should be given to the mother?

Anne should be told that factor VIII replacement therapy will stop the bleeding and with appropriate treatment her child should have a normal life expectancy.

PART 2: CASES

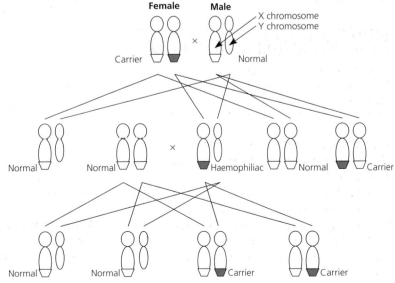

Figure 118 X-linked inheritance. Three chromosomes are shown: a normal X (tip of long arm unshaded), an X-bearing a mutant factor VIII gene (tip of long arm shaded) and a normal Y. A female carrier with a normal partner has four types of offspring with equal frequency: normal son, haemophiliac son, normal daughter and carrier daughter. A haemophiliac male has only two types of offspring: carrier daughters and normal sons.

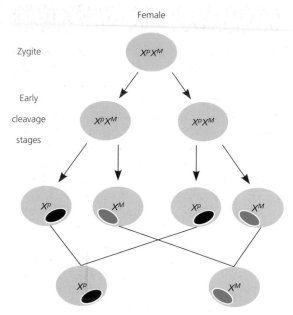

Female

Zygite

Early cleavage stages

Figure 119 Lyonization (after Mary Lyon) is the name given to the process of inactivation of one member of the pair of X chromosomes in every female cell. It occurs in all somatic cells of the female embryo on the 16th day after fertilization when it comprises around 5000 cells. For any somatic cell the choice as to whether paternal (X^P) or the maternal (X^M) X chromosome is inactivated is random (the inactive X is shown as a dark mass). Hence, normal females are mosaics with a mixture of X^M and X^P. Because of the intrinsic randomness of the inactivation process, the relative proportions of gene–protein expression vary from female to female. This accounts for the variable expression of X-linked recessive traits in heterozygous females, who may be symptomatic if most cells are utilizing the defective gene on the X chromosome.

> **KEY POINT**
>
> Bleeding must be treated promptly and appropriately. The dose of FVIII replacement is determined by its volume of distribution, the half-life and the haemostatic requirement of the type of bleeding. Haemarthroses and soft tissue bleeds require 50% correction while life-threatening haemorrhages require 80–100%. Prophylactic use of concentrates, which prevent severe bleeding, is now commonly recommended. Life threatening bleeding should always be treated with 100% correction.

Figure 120 shows a chronic knee haemarthrosis. Muscle wasting in the quadriceps is evident.

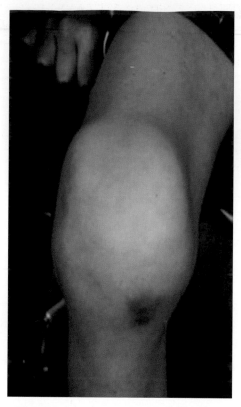

Figure 120 A chronic knee haemarthrosis (bleeding into the knee joint) with marked quadriceps muscle wasting. This should be a rare occurrence with proper therapy and prophylaxis.

From where is factor VIII concentrate derived?

Factor VIII concentrates are made from human plasma or from genetically engineered mammalian cells.

What risks does the administration of a concentrate from human plasma carry?

The administration of blood products made from human plasma always carries the potential risk of transmitting viral or other infections. However, the combination of strict donor viral screening protocols and intensive donor self-exclusion programmes together with viral inactivation processes have prevented HIV or hepatitis C transmission from the use of plasma-derived factor concentrates since the late 1980s. These viral inactivation steps are not effective against parvovirus B19, hepatitis A or Creutzfeldt–Jakob prions.

KEY POINT

Recombinant coagulation factor products offer the best possible protection from transmission of human blood-borne viruses and are regarded as the treatment of choice for all patients with haemophilia.

Can you now construct an algorithm to investigate a baby who has a bleed shortly after delivery?

Yes.

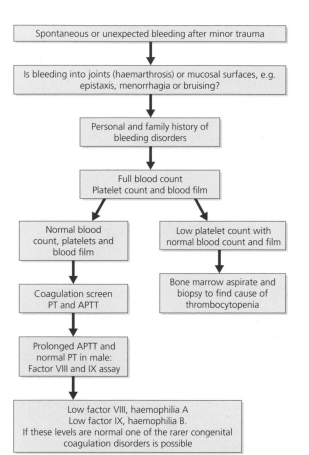

The baby was treated with recombinant FVIII (25 IU/kg) intravenously twice daily for 3 days. Cranial ultrasound showed no evidence of intraventricular haemorrhage. The child was subsequently referred to a paediatric haemophilia centre where he attended every 3 months. At the age of 18 months prophylactic replacement therapy was commenced because of a severe bleed into his knee joint.

CASE REVIEW

The birth of a baby should be, and usually is, a joyous occasion. The possibility of a serious congenital disorder is something that many women fear and it is a difficult task to explain such a probable diagnosis at such an emotional time. However, it is important to recognize a serious problem and call for help quickly. Although it may be a traumatic occasion for the mother it is more difficult if the diagnosis is missed or made much later.

Access to rapid blood analysis and specialist opinion has made early diagnosis easier. In the case of congenital deficiency of factor VIII or IX a family history is very helpful if it is positive. The major question arises with the sister of a known person with haemophilia. Because factor VIII and IX are X-linked diseases remember that the affected person's sister may or may not be a carrier but the daughter of a person with haemophilia is always a carrier. As explained, spontaneous mutations may occur without a bleeding history.

The early diagnosis in this case was suspected after the initial coagulation screen and confirmed by factor assay.

Factor XI deficiency is found predominantly in Ashkenazi Jews but clinical manifestations are highly variable. In some cases bleeding following circumcision may be the initial clue.

Referral to an expert centre is required to plan treatment and to review the patient at regular intervals.

KEY POINTS

- The modern history of haemophilia has been extremely uncertain. Over the last 30 years the disease has gone from one in which joint deformity and premature death were not uncommon to a situation where factor V replacement was commonly available and the morbidity and mortality completely changed. This happy period was brought to a sad and abrupt end with the transmission of HIV infection through human factor concentrates. Many lives were lost and trust in the medical system in many countries was eroded
- The combination of widespread publicity, intrusive history-taking from prospective plasma donors and the development of good screening tests for viral illnesses combined to make plasma derived factor concentrates safer. The introduction of methods to inactivate viruses

Continued

in plasma-derived products and subsequently the manufacture of recombinant concentrates has restored confidence in the medical system and once again improved the quality of life of patients with factor VIII or IX deficiency
- Unfortunately, high costs make the provision of recombinant factor concentrates unavailable to many patients worldwide
- In some countries, antenatal screening of fetuses with possible factor VIII or IX deficiency has been instituted to try to reduce the 'gene pool'

Further reading

Arceci RJ, Hann IM & Smith OP. *Paediatric Haematology*. Blackwell Publishing, Oxford, 2006.

Colman RW, Hirsh J, Marder VJ, Clowes AW & George JN, eds. *Haemostasis and Thrombosis: Basic Principles and Clinical Practice*, 4th edn. Lippincott William & Wilkin, 2001.

Kitchens CS, Alving BM & Kessler CM, eds. *Consultative Haemostasis and Thrombosis*. WB Saunders, 2002.

DiMichele D. Hemophilia 1996: new approach to an old disease. *Pediatric Clinics of North America* 1996; **43**: 709–736.

World Federation of Haemophilia: www.wfh.org Accessed in Dec 2006.

A 26-year-old woman with chest pain following a long aeroplane journey

Six hours following her return from Australia to Copenhagen, Eva Strinberg, a 26-year-old pharmacist, developed chest pain. The chest pain was predominantly right sided. It was so severe and she was very distressed she requested her family doctor to come to her home.

What is the differential diagnosis?

Sudden onset of severe chest pain in a young adult suggests a pneumothorax (collapsed lung). There are usually no prodromal events and the pain may be severe. Pneumonia can cause chest pain and distress but is usually preceded by a cough and fever. Myocardial infarction or a dissecting aortic aneurysm could cause the symptoms but would be very unlikely in such a young girl. A pulmonary embolus is possible, especially in view of the recent history of a long aeroplane flight (see key point, p. 135).

What should the family doctor do?

Arrange to have Eva taken to the nearest accident and emergency (A&E) department.

What should be done on arrival at the A&E department?

A full history and physical examination should be carried out.

What aspects of the history should the doctor in the A&E department concentrate upon?

A history of any previous similar episode or leg swelling. A family history of similar complaints. The doctor would be looking for clues to a hypercoagulable state in the patient or her family.

Haematology: Clinical Cases Uncovered. By S. McCann, R. Foà, O. Smith and E. Conneally. Published 2009 by Blackwell Publishing, ISBN: 978-1-4051-8322-2

Physical examination was unremarkable apart from the reduced air entry in her right mid lung region and her chest pain was made worse on deep inspiration. Eva was hypoxaemic (O_2 saturation 90% on room air; normal >96%).

Now what is the differential diagnosis?

Pulmonary embolism (PE) is likely in view of the history, paucity of other physical signs and hypoxaemia. A large spontaneous pneumothorax could present in the same way.

What should be done next?

A chest radiograph, coagulation screen (Table 54) and an electrocardiograph (ECG).

The chest radiograph was normal and the ECG showed a sinus tachycardia.

How do the chest radiographic findings, ECG and coagulation results help to confirm your suspicion of a PE?

Neither the ECG nor the chest radiograph point to a specific diagnosis and the coagulation screen is normal.

What further test should be performed to make the diagnosis?

D-dimers should be assayed in Eva's plasma. A computed tomography (CT) pulmonary angiogram should be carried out.

The CT angiogram (Fig. 121) shows defects consistent with an embolus (arrows) in the pulmonary circulation (PE).

Now what is the differential diagnosis?

A pneumothorax is not identified radiologically and there is no evidence of infection. This makes the diagnosis of PE very likely.

Table 54 Results of the coagulation screen.

Tests	Patient's result	Normal range
PT	13 s	11–14 s
APTT	40 s	31–44 s

APTT, activated partial thromboplastin time; PT, prothrombin time.

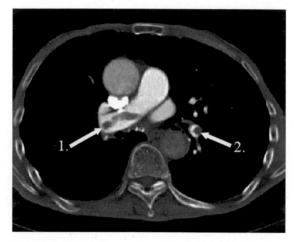

Figure 121 Computed tomography (CT) angiogram showing a filling defect consistent with a pulmonary embolus (arrows).

What should be done next?

Eva should be given oxygen support, adequate pain relief and anticoagulation with heparin. Heparin is available in unfractionated or low molecular weight forms (LMWH).

How can a normal coagulation screen be reconciled with a PE in an otherwise healthy young patient?

Inherited prothrombotic states (thrombophilia) may dispose to venous thrombosis and/or emboli (VTE) with a normal coagulation screen. Prolonged times in cramped positions may predispose to VTE (see key point, p. 135).

What further blood test will help to confirm if an embolus has occurred?

D-dimer measurement (Table 55).

How can the elevated D-dimers be explained?

D-dimers are elevated in the plasma following the conversion of fibrinogen to fibrin during clot formation

Table 55 Result of D-dimer test.

	Patient's results	Normal values
D-dimer	6000 µg/mL	<200 µg/mL

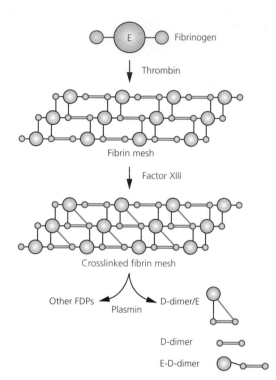

Figure 122 Structure of D-dimers in the plasma. Generation of cross-linked fibrin by thrombin and factor XIII. Plasmin degrades cross-linked fibrin to fibrin degradation products and D-dimers.

and their subsequent breakdown of fibrin by plasmin (Fig. 122). This finding is consistent with a diagnosis of PE.

How could the family history help to determine if Eva has a prothrombotic state?

It is common to find a history of embolism in first degree relatives.

KEY POINT

Many prothrombotic states are inherited and are often caused by single mutations of proteins in the anticoagulant pathway.

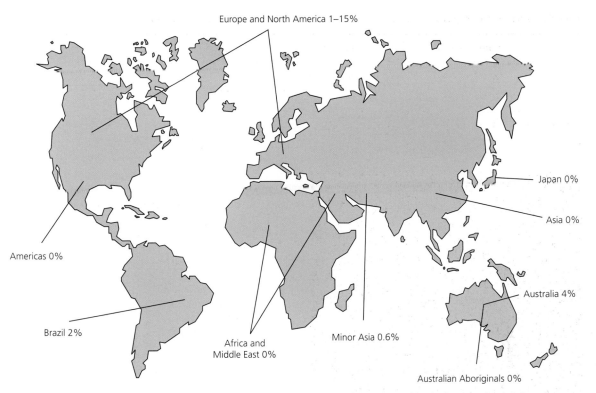

Figure 123 Factor V Leiden allele is found only in Caucasians and the prevalence of this polymorphism in the general population of Western societies has considerable variation. High prevalence (up to 15%) is found in southern Sweden, Germany, Greece and Israel. In the Netherlands, UK, Ireland and the USA around 3–5% of the population carry the mutant alleles. Lower prevalence of around 2% is found in Hispanics.

What further questions should be asked to assess other risk factors for embolism in a young woman?

Eva should be asked about smoking, oral contraceptives and her ethnic background (Fig. 123). Women of child-bearing age should also be asked about a history of recurrent spontaneous abortion, intrauterine growth retardation and pre-eclampsia.

Eva had been taking oral contraceptives for 3 years and two of her first cousins developed clots in their leg veins during and after pregnancy.

KEY POINT

VTE that happen following long-haul air flights have been given the name 'economy class syndrome'. This results from sitting in a cramped position without adequate exercise and probable dehydration accentuated by alcohol ingestion. However, most patients who have the 'economy class syndrome' have risk factors for venous thrombosis.

Table 56 Inherited thrombophilia.

Type of abnormality	Investigations
Protein C deficiency	Clotting test
Protein S deficiency	Clotting test
Factor V Leiden	Clotting test and genetic test
Prothrombin G202 10A	Genetic test

How might you investigate what types of inherited coagulation disorder can give rise to prothrombotic states?

Look for inherited deficiencies of proteins C and S and polymorphisms of factor V or prothrombin. These inherited deficiencies can be measured by more sophisticated clotting assays or by genetic tests (Table 56).

Further investigation revealed factor V Leiden (the most common coagulation factor variant leading to a prothrombotic state). These inherited abnormalities are called thrombophilia.

What advantage does LMWH have over unfractionated heparin when treating Eva?

LMWH has a long plasma half-life and a more predictable dose–response, making monitoring with blood tests unnecessary other than in pregnancy and renal failure.

For how long should anticoagulation be continued after initial heparinization?

The anticoagulant warfarin can be started within 24 hours of the heparin treatment and should be continued for 6 months.

> **KEY POINT**
>
> Women with thrombophilia who use the oral contraceptive pill (OCP) develop blood clots more often and sooner after initiation of the OCP than women without thrombophilia.

How would you consider carrying out population studies to detect inherited thrombophilia?

It is practical only in young women with a family history of thromboses or known thrombophilia.

What method of contraception should Eva be advised to use?

Barrier methods or medroxyprogesterone (a depo injection every 3 months).

What advice should be given to Eva before undertaking long flights or journeys?

She should be advised to wear support stockings, exercise hourly and refrain from alcohol.

What drug could be used as prophylaxis against VTE?

LMWH given shortly before the flight.

> **KEY POINT**
>
> Aspirin has been recommended but would be totally ineffectual in preventing VTE and may cause gastric irritation and bleeding (Case 17).

Can you now construct an algorithm for a young girl with sudden onset of severe chest pain?

Yes.

A previously healthy young girl with sudden onset of chest pain
Tachycardia and hypoxaemia; normal chest X-ray
FBC. Look for high platelet count or evidence of haematological malignancy
CT pulmonary angiogram. Evidence of PE
Positive CT angio Treat heparin/warfarin Treat with fibrinolytic agents if PE is life-threatening
Investigate for underlying cause, e.g. cancer, thrombophilia
If thrombophilia screen positive consider screening first degree relatives

Outcome. Eva was commenced on LMWH at therapeutic doses without monitoring. She was sent home the next day after commencing warfarin with daily monitoring. She was treated for 6 months. A year later Eva became pregnant and was given prophylactic LMWH. Given her history of VTE and FV Leiden, prophylactic LMWH was administered throughout her pregnancy and for a further 6 weeks postpartum with no recurrence of thrombotic episodes. Both of her cousins were heterozygous for the FV Leiden polymorphism.

CASE REVIEW

A young woman presents with sudden onset chest pain and severe distress. Clearly, she has a medical problem and her symptoms are unlikely to be caused by anxiety alone. It is important to get her expert medical assessment immediately as she cannot be assessed adequately in a family doctor setting.

In this case there are two important issues. First, to take a full history and, secondly, to make the correct diagnosis quickly.

This woman gives a history of prolonged travel which is the clue. This story, combined with her symptoms and physical signs, make the diagnosis of PE likely. It is important to make the diagnosis rapidly as the treatment outcome will be better with early treatment.

The investigation that is most likely to give you the correct diagnosis is a pulmonary CT angiogram. A ventilation/perfusion scan is useful if CT angiogram is not available.

KEY POINTS

- There is significant public awareness of deep vein thrombosis in recent years
- There is widespread discussion about VTE following prolonged travel. A case has been made for aspirin prophylaxis but if any prophylaxis was considered it should be a single administration of LMWH. However, this requires an injection which is impractical for most travellers. Widespread use of aspirin will lead to some cases of severe gastrointestinal bleeding and in risk–benefit analysis has not been shown to be justified
- In patients with high risk, e.g. cancer, known thrombophilia with a prior VTE and/or taking OCP, gross obesity and heavy cigarette smoking, LMWH should be considered with elastic stockings and mobilization

Further reading

Colman RW, Hirsh J, Marder VJ, Clowes AW & George JN, eds. *Haemostasis and Thrombosis: Basic Principles and Clinical Practice*, 5th edn. Lippincott William & Wilkin, 2007.

Heit JA. Thrombophilia. asheducationbook.hematologylibrary. org/cgi/content/full/2007/1/127 Accessed in 2007.

Hoffbrand AV, Moss PAH & Pettit JE. *Essential Haematology*, 5th edn. Blackwell Publishing, 2006: 303–319.

Khoury MJ, McCabe LL & McCabe ERB. Population screening in the age of genomic medicine. *New England Journal of Medicine* 2003; **348**: 50–58.

Kinane TB, Grabowski EF, Sharma A, Nimkin K, King ME & Cornell LD. Case records of the Massachusetts General Hopital. Case 7-2008: a 17-year-old girl with chest pain and haemoptysis. *New England Journal of Medicine* 2008; **358**: 941–952.

Kitchens CS, Alving BM, Kessler CM, eds. *Consultative Haemostasis and Thrombosis*. WB Saunders, 2007.

Case 20 A 27-year-old woman afraid to receive a blood transfusion

Lai Ching-te, a 27-year-old schoolteacher, was involved in a road traffic accident. Lai was taken to the nearest accident and emergency department. She was found to have a fractured pelvis, a compound fracture of her right femur and a laceration on her face. Lai was started on intravenous fluids and the laceration was sutured. She was then transferred to the orthopaedic team for further management.

A history revealed that Lai had never been in hospital before. She was not taking any medications. She was married but had no children. Lai did not smoke or drink alcohol.

On examination in the surgical unit Lai appeared pale and sweaty and her BP was 80/50 mmHg and pulse 110 beats/minute.

Laboratory investigations revealed the information in Table 57. The blood film showed polychromasia (Fig. 124).

What is the explanation for the blood findings?

The anaemia is probably caused by blood loss. The polychromasia reflects an increased number of reticulocytes. The word 'polychromasia' refers to the blue–grey colour of these cells, which reflects the ribosomal content. The slightly raised neutrophil and platelet count are a response to the bleeding. A large number of platelets are normally present in the spleen. Following major trauma they are released into the circulation, accounting for the rise in the platelet count.

How should this patient be managed?

Lai will require a general anaesthetic for surgical fixation of her fractures.

Haematology: Clinical Cases Uncovered. By S. McCann, R. Foà, O. Smith and E. Conneally. Published 2009 by Blackwell Publishing, ISBN: 978-1-4051-8322-2

Why might she require blood transfusion?

Her haemoglobin is <8.0 g/dL and Lai has evidence of active bleeding as measured by her vital signs (BP and pulse).

Although intravenous fluids are used to correct hypovolaemic 'shock', the rapid onset of anaemia in this case may lead to insufficient oxygen delivery to the tissues which is an indication for red cell transfusion.

There is no absolute haemoglobin at which blood transfusion is indicated, a 'transfusion trigger' of 7.0 g/dL in a previously healthy young patient is commonly taken as the level at which transfusion is necessary to preserve tissue oxygenation. The decision to recommend blood transfusion will depend on the cause and speed of onset of the anaemia as well as the patient's age and general health. Anaemia that is gradual in onset is often well tolerated by the patient and if the underlying cause is corrected a blood transfusion may not be necessary.

> **KEY POINT**
>
> Red cells are transfused to maintain tissue oxygenation and prevent hypoxia, not to treat hypovolaemia or maintain a 'normal' haemoglobin.

How might you respond if the patient says: 'Doctor, will I get an infection from the blood?'

Tell her that if she bleeds further it is safer to have a blood transfusion than run the risks caused by ongoing blood loss.

> **KEY POINT**
>
> Transfusion of any blood product will always carry the risk of transmitting an infectious agent.

Table 57 Results of the full blood count.

	Patient's results	Normal range
Hb	7.0 g/dL	11.5–16.4 g/dL
MCV	96 fL	83.0–99.0 fL (μm³)
WBC	12.0 × 10⁹/L	4.0–11.0 × 10⁹/L (10³/μL)
Neutrophils	10.0 × 10⁹/L	2.0–7.5 × 10⁹/L (10³/μL)
Lymphocytes	2.0 × 10⁹/L	1.5–3.5 × 10⁹/L (10³/μL)
Platelets	500 × 10⁹/L	140–450 × 10⁹/L (10³/μL)

Hb, haemoglobin; MCV, mean corpuscular haemoglobin; WBC, white blood cell count.

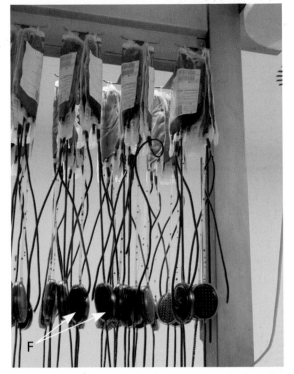

Figure 125 White cells being removed by filtration from whole blood.

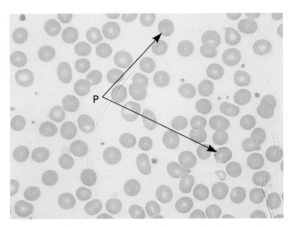

Figure 124 Blood film showing polychromasia (P).

Previously, transmission of HIV via blood and blood products (especially clotting factor concentrates) resulted in human tragedy, with illness and death for many patients. Transmission occurred before the virus had been identified. Blood and blood products transmitted hepatitis C virus (HCV), again before the virus had been identified. Malaria can also be transmitted and, more recently, West Nile virus has been transmitted by blood transfusion. It has also been established that new variant Creutzfeldt–Jakob disease (vCJD) can be transmitted by blood transfusion.

To minimize the possibility of prion transmission (vCJD) and to reduce the number of febrile transfusion reactions, white cells can be removed (leucodepletion) from blood after collection (Fig. 125).

What has changed in the world of blood transfusion to make blood and blood products safer?

Careful screening and testing of blood donors, and where feasible treatment of blood to remove infectious agents:

1 Use of volunteer non-remunerated donors wherever possible.

2 Careful screening of all blood donors including a detailed history and a number of intrusive questions about sexual history and substance abuse (Table 58).

3 A detailed travel history from donors who have recently visited an area where a particular disease or virus is endemic, e.g. tropical areas for malaria, USA for West Nile virus. Volunteers are not permitted to donate until the incubation period is past. In some cases the donor may be permanently excluded from donating, e.g. extended UK residence during the risk period for vCJD, or residence as a child in a malaria area or in

Table 58 An example of questions asked of a potential donor. From the Irish Blood Transfusion Service Donor Health Questionnaire.

1 Are you giving bloods to be tested for HIV/AIDS or hepatitis?

2 Have you **ever** injected or been injected with non-prescription drugs – **even once or a long time ago?** This includes bodybuilding drugs.

3 If you are a male, have you **ever** had oral or anal sex with another male – even if a condom or other protection was used?

4 Have you **ever** received money or drugs for sex?

5 Do you or your partner have HIV/AIDS?

6 Do you or your partner or close household contacts have hepatitis B or C?

If the answer to any of the above is YES, or if you are in any doubt, you must indicate YES, and NOT donate

rural South and Central America for Chaga's disease (trypanosomiasis).

4 Laboratory testing of donated blood for antibodies to known viruses: HIV, hepatitis B virus (HBV) and HCV. More recently testing for nucleic acid sequences (NAT) for the above viruses is available.

5 White cell removal which may remove or reduce pathogens, e.g. viruses, intracellular bacteria, parasites or prions.

6 Plasma and blood products such as coagulation concentrates can be virally inactivated. Methods to treat platelets are becoming available. Currently, it is not possible to apply these techniques to red blood cell transfusions.

7 In some countries widespread public campaigns making people aware of the dangers of donating if they are possibly infected with one of the viruses mentioned.

8 Making sure those new donors are screened on two occasions before blood is taken for transfusion.

How has the introduction of these measures made a difference in terms of safety of blood transfusion?

Donor history screening and testing of donations has markedly reduced the risk of transmitting disease by blood transfusion.

Table 59 Estimated frequency of transmitting viral infections from blood.

Hepatitis B*	1 in 250,000
HIV	1 in 8 million
HCV	1 in 30 million

*Although the estimate is 1 in 250,000, the actual incidence seems to be much lower and with widespread use of new tests will be significantly less than 1 in 250,000.

> **KEY POINT**
>
> The risk of transmitting known viruses is now so low that it cannot be quantified and must be estimated using mathematical models (Table 59).

What is meant by a 'window period'?

A 'lag' period, after a viral infection, before antibodies are produced in the infected individual.

> **KEY POINT**
>
> If the transfusion service is testing donors for antibodies it is possible that an infected donor could be 'missed' as the donation might be taken after a viral infection and before the antibodies can be detected. The introduction of NAT will detect the virus immediately after infection.

What do the terms 'blood components' and 'blood products' mean?

Blood contains cells (red cells, white cells and platelets) and liquid (plasma) in which proteins and clotting factors are present (Table 60; Figs 126–129).

Before requesting blood for this patient what further information is required?

Lai should be asked about a past history of blood transfusion and pregnancies, even if they had ended prematurely, naturally or by abortion.

Why are these questions important?

Antibodies may be formed to antigens on the transfused or fetal red cells. Red blood cells have over 200 antigens, which are expressed on the cell surface. Only the ABO and RhD group antigens are matched for prior to

Table 60 Blood components and products.

Red cells	When blood is collected from a donor it is centrifuged, the white cells are removed by filtration and the platelets and plasma are saved for further use (Fig. 126). The red cells are suspended in a preservative solution and can be used for up to 27–42 days depending on the preservative solution. Currently, red cells cannot be treated to inactivate viruses
Platelets	Platelets for transfusion may be separated from blood at the time of collection and suspended in plasma until they are ready for use (up to 5 days). Alternatively, the donor may be attached to a machine where blood is continuously centrifuged and a large number of platelets removed and stored for transfusion (Fig. 127). The red blood cells and plasma are returned to the donor. This is called platelet pheresis and is equivalent to individual collections from four donors. Methods of viral inactivation for platelets have been developed and are currently coming into use
Plasma	Plasma can be collected from individual units of blood (Fig. 128) or collected by plasma pheresis. Plasma can be frozen and stored for 2 years before use. Plasma can be treated to inactivate viruses
Blood products Factor 'concentrates'	Blood products are manufactured from plasma 'pooled' from large numbers of donors. Albumin, factors VIII, IX, VII and fibrinogen can be made into 'concentrates' for replacement therapy (Fig. 129). All these 'concentrates' can be treated to inactivate viruses Because of the possibility of transmitting viral infections from plasma from large donor pools, so-called 'recombinant' products are also available. These recombinant products are manufactured by transfecting animal 'cell lines' with the human gene for the particular factor required, e.g. factor VIII gene into Chinese hamster ovary cells

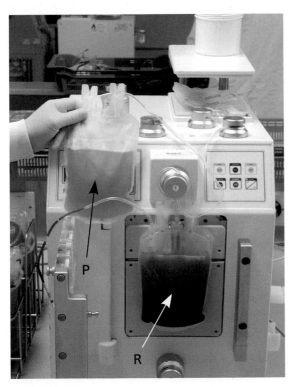

Figure 126 Preparation of red cells for transfusion. Plasma (P) is removed and red cells (R) suspended in a preservative solution.

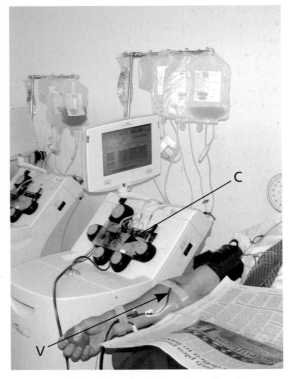

Figure 127 Platelets being collected by centrifugation. C, centrifuge; V, vein.

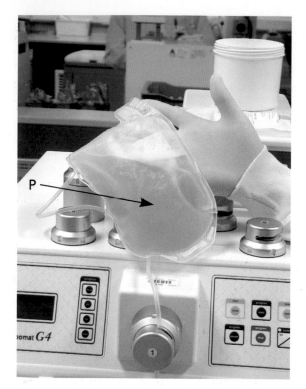

Figure 128 Plasma (P) before freezing.

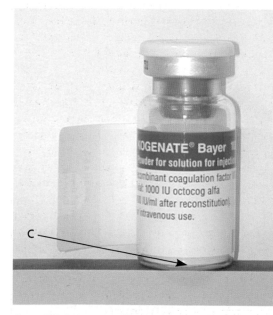

Figure 129 Concentrate of factor VIII (C).

transfusion. If a patient receives red cells with other antigens that are different from the antigens on the patient's own red cells, he/she may make antibodies to these foreign antigens. These antibodies may not cause a problem and may be present in small amounts in the patient's blood. If at a future date another blood transfusion is given with the same foreign antigens on the red cells, a 'haemolytic' transfusion reaction may take place where the antibodies in the patient's blood attack the transfused red blood cells. This can result in destruction of all the transfused cells, and rarely renal failure (non-ABO acute transfusion reactions are very rarely fatal).

These questions are important if the laboratory finds that Lai's sample reacts in the antibody screening test or in the cross-match and may delay provision of compatible blood. If she has received a prior blood transfusion she should be asked if she was told she had developed antibodies.

> **KEY POINT**
>
> At the time of delivery or abortion, red cells from the fetus may cross into the mother's circulation. The mother may make antibodies (fetal red cells have antigens from both parents). Future blood transfusion may cause similar problems.

What features of pregnancy and red cell antigens could cause further problems?

Antibodies can cross the placenta from the mother and cause haemolysis in the fetus. An RhD negative mother who has a RhD positive baby may develop anti-D antibodies after the pregnancy or more rarely during pregnancy. These antibodies may increase in amount in the mother's circulation in subsequent pregnancies and cross the placenta (this time in the opposite direction) from the mother to the fetus and cause destruction of the fetal red cells causing haemolytic disease of the newborn.

What other precautions are taken prior to blood transfusion?

The patient must have a sample taken for ABO and RhD grouping and screening for possible antibodies, which might be present from a previous transfusion or pregnancy, to allow correctly matched blood to be provided. The patient must be asked to identify themselves ('Please state your name and DOB', not 'Are you Mrs Murphy?'; Part 1) and the details checked against the patient's ID band. If these match the sample is taken and must be labelled at the bedside. Electronic systems using bar code identification (similar to the supermarket) can be used to check the identity of the patient and the blood for donation.

In an emergency when the patient requires blood before a sample can be tested, O Rh negative blood can be transfused. (A stock of checked emergency O Rh negative blood should be available in the hospital.)

What might go wrong?

Human error. The most common cause of a blood transfusion problem is human mistake, e.g. failure to identify the patient at sampling leading to the blood sample taken from wrong patient or failing to check the identity of patient and unit at administration so the wrong blood is given to the patient or the blood is given to the wrong patient.

Can you construct an algorithm for safe blood transfusion?

Yes.

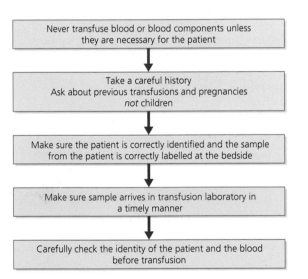

Outcome. Lai received 3 units of blood prior to and during surgery which was uneventful. Her postoperative haemoglobin was 9.5 g/dL and she was given iron tablets. Lai was discharged from hospital 3 weeks later and attended the physiotherapy department until she had fully recovered. Her haemoglobin was 12.5 g/dL on discharge but she was advised to continue iron tablets for a further 3 months to replace her iron stores. Two years later Lai became pregnant. Antenatal screening for red cell antibodies was negative and Lai had a normal healthy baby.

Some religious beliefs forbid the use of blood transfusion (e.g. Jehovah's Witnesses). With careful management, cardiac surgery, organ transplantation and even haematological diseases such as leukaemia have been successfully treated without the use of blood transfusions.

CASE REVIEW

Since the transmission of HIV and HCV infection through blood transfusion there has been a considerable loss of trust by the public about the safety of blood transfusions. This was compounded by the transmission of HIV, a fatal infection at the time, to many thousands of patients with factor VIII and IX deficiency via factor concentrates derived from human plasma. Much suffering and many deaths happened and pressure was applied to transfusion services and pharmaceutical companies to provide safe blood and blood products.

Many strange ideas developed such as it is possible to contract HIV by donating blood. The position of trust made it very difficult for many transfusion services to obtain adequate supplies of blood during the late 1980s and early 1990s. Many patients in hospital are fearful of receiving blood or blood products and the question asked by our patient is a common one.

Thankfully, the risk of viral or other pathogen transmission has been greatly reduced by donor screening, universal leucodepletion and viral inactivation whenever possible. As yet there is no safe way to 'inactivate' red cell concentrates so we depend on accurate history-taking from the donor, high-quality screening and quality controlled antibody and in some cases NAT.

A more conservative approach to transfusion has been taken and blood transfusion is not given unless it is required. In some cases one unit of red cells may suffice, a practice that was frowned upon 15 years ago. Elective surgical interventions have been critically evaluated and blood usage has been successfully reduced without compromising the patient's outcome.

KEY POINTS

- Technology has made blood and blood transfusion safer
- Pharmaceutical companies use 'state of the art' technology
- Blood transfusion centres use unpaid volunteer donors
- Some pharmaceutical companies use paid donors for repeated plasma donations but scrutinize them carefully and use the best inactivation methods to prevent spread of infectious agents
- Recombinant technology to manufacture some factor concentrates avoids the use of human plasma but the products are very costly
- Platelet transfusions are usually reserved for patients in whom the risk of bleeding is believed to be imminent. Traditionally, platelet transfusions were given when the count went below 20×10^9/L but this figure has been subsequently reduced to 10×10^9/L or less in some institutions. The decision to transfuse platelets requires significant experience and knowledge and should be taken by senior physicians. As in red cell transfusion, the decision to transfuse platelets will be guided by the clinical state of the patient, coexisting diseases and medications especially those interfering with platelet function
- The requirement for platelet transfusions in immune-mediated thrombocytopenia is rare (Case 17)
- Remember, the majority of serious 'transfusion reactions' are caused by human error

Further reading

Bracer AW, Schlicter SJ, Stanworth SJ & Hess JR. Transfusion medicine. asheducationbook.hematologylibrary.org/cgi/content/full/2007/ Accessed in 2007.

Hoffbrand AV, Moss PAH & Pettit JE. *Essential Haematology*, 5th edn. Blackwell Publishing, Oxford, 2006: 337–351.

Lundy D, Lasoina S, Kaplan H, Rabin-Fastman B, Lawlor E. Seven hundred and fifty-nine chances to learn: a 3-year pilot project to analyse transfusion-related near-miss events in the Republic of Ireland. *Vox Sang* 2007; **92**: 233–241.

Mazza P, Prudenzano A, Amurri B, Palazzo G, Pisapia G, Stani L *et al*. Myeloablative therapy and bone marrow transplantation in Jehovah's Witnesses with malignancies: single centre experience. *Bone Marrow Transplantation* 2003; **32**: 433–436.

Prowse CV. An ABC for West Nile virus. *Transfusion Medicine* 2003; **13**: 1–7.

Soldan K, Barbara JAJ, Ramsay ME & Hall AJ. Estimation of the risk of hepatitis B virus, hepatitis C virus and human immunodeficiency virus infectious donations entering the blood supply in England, 1993–2001. *Vox Sanguinis* 2003; **84**: 274–286.

Case 21 A 35-year-old woman with an elevated platelet count

Maria Kazantzakis, a 35-year-old IT consultant was referred to her family doctor because she was found to have a high platelet count when she went to donate blood. Maria complained of fatigue and a headache for about 6 months. She was diagnosed with essential hypertension 5 years previously and was on treatment with atenolol. Maria's headache was severe and generalized. There were no precipitating or relieving factors. There were no associated features and it was partially relieved by paracetamol.

What is your differential diagnosis?

A high platelet count is found in a number of conditions such as chronic inflammatory diseases, following a bleed, with metastatic cancer, polycythaemia vera (PV), chronic myeloid leukaemia (CML), some myelodysplastic diseases (MDS), following splenectomy and essential thrombocythaemia (ET).

What should be done next?

A full history and physical examination.

There was nothing else relevant in Maria's history. Her fatigue caused her to miss her aerobic classes for the previous 3 months. Maria did not smoke and consumed 14 units/week alcohol. Her only medication was atenolol 50 mg/day. There was no family history of blood diseases. Her mother was alive but her father had died at the age of 55 from a myocardial infarction. Maria's two siblings were alive and she had no pregnancies or children. She had been married to an engineer for 3 years. There were no abnormal physical findings. Her blood pressure was 125/80 mmHg and her fundi were normal.

Haematology: Clinical Cases Uncovered. By S. McCann, R. Foà, O. Smith and E. Conneally. Published 2009 by Blackwell Publishing, ISBN: 978-1-4051-8322-2

What should the family doctor do next?

Blood should be sent to the nearest laboratory for a full blood count (see Table 61) and a blood film should be requested. Maria should be told to return for the result in 2 days.

The blood film was reported as showing a marked increase in platelets with platelet anisocytosis and poikilocytosis. The red cells and white cells appeared normal.

Now what is your differential diagnosis?

The high platelet count is verified and the abnormal sized and shaped platelets are in keeping with a diagnosis of ET (Fig. 130). There is no history of a bleed and the platelet count would not be expected to reach this level following haemorrhage. There is nothing in the history to suggest cancer (her breast and rectal examination was normal) or a chronic inflammatory disorder. CML and MDS are unlikely because of the absence of white cell precursors, a normal white cell count and a normal appearance of the neutrophils in the blood film.

KEY POINT

Many patients with high platelet counts are identified by blood counts in the absence of symptoms. However, the common presenting symptoms are headache, erythromelalgia (burning pain usually in feet caused by microvascular occlusion, commonly with pre-existing peripheral vascular disease), transient ischaemic attacks (TIAs), leg vein thrombosis and gastrointestinal bleeding.

Signs are those of the bleeding defect or thrombosis but are non-specific. An enlarged spleen is found in about 40% of patients.

What should be done next?

In view of the potentially serious diagnosis, Maria should be told she probably has a blood disease and needs a specialist opinion.

Table 61 Results of the blood tests.

	Patient's results	Normal range
Hb	14 g/dL	11.5–16.4 g/dL
MCV	90 fL	83–99 fL (μm^3)
MCH	30 pg/cell	26.7–32.5 pg/cell
MCHC	32 g/dL	30.8–34.6 g/dL
RBC	5.0×10^{12}/L	$4.00–5.20 \times 10^{12}$/L (10^6/μL)
WBC	8.5×10^9/L	$4.0–11.0 \times 10^9$/L (10^3/μL)
Platelets	1413×10^9/L	$150–450 \times 10^9$/L (10^3/μL)

Hb, haemoglobin; MCH, mean corpuscular haemoglobin; MCHC, mean corpuscular haemoglobin concentration; MCV, mean corpuscular volume; RBC, red blood cell count; WBC, white blood cell count.

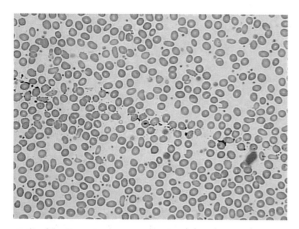

Figure 130 Blood film with large and abnormally shaped platelets.

She was given an appointment with a haematologist for the following day.

What medication should be considered in the interval?

Aspirin 75 mg/day, with meals, should be prescribed.

> **KEY POINT**
>
> Patients with elevated platelet counts >1000 × 10^9/L are in danger of thrombosis and/or bleeding and may benefit from aspirin. Microvascular occlusion may respond rapidly to aspirin.

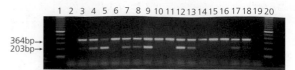

Figure 131 DNA analysis of *JAK2* kinase mutations. DNA is extracted from whole blood and is subjected to an allele-specific polymerase chain reaction (PCR) which identifies a control band (364 bp) in all patient samples and a smaller band (203 bp) in those patients in whom the *JAK2* V617F is present. Lanes 1 and 20 contain a DNA ladder; lanes 2 and 19, PCR negative controls; lanes 3 and 18, PCR positive controls; lanes 4–9, polycythaemia vera (PV) patients; lanes 10–13, essential thrombocythaemia (ET) patients; lanes 14–17, primary myelofibrosis (PMF) patients.

What should the haematologist do?

Repeat the history and physical exam and look at the blood film.

What further investigations should be ordered?

A biochemical screen, a chest radiograph and an ultrasound examination of the abdomen to assess spleen size.

The biochemical screen, chest radiograph and ultrasound examination were normal.

What specific test should be carried out to confirm if the diagnosis is ET or if there is some other cause for the elevated platelet count?

A molecular test for the *JAK2* kinase mutation. As can be seen from Fig. 131, kinase mutation is only found in 50% of cases of ET. Therefore, if the test is positive it confirms the diagnosis in the appropriate clinical setting. A negative test is unhelpful and the clinician is still left with the possibility of other diagnoses. A cytogenetic analysis and/or fluorescence *in situ* hybridization (FISH) should be undertaken to exclude a diagnosis of CML (Case 10).

The cytogenetic and FISH analyses were normal. As the *JAK* kinase mutation was not found in this case, what further investigation should now be undertaken?

A bone marrow aspirate and biopsy should be carried out (Figs 132 and 133).

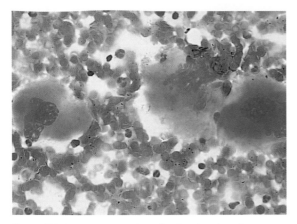

Figure 132 Bone marrow aspirate showing clumping of megakaryocytes.

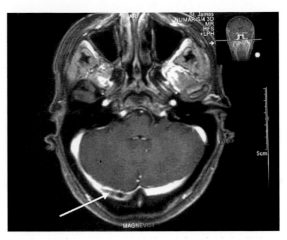

Figure 134 Contrast enhanced magnetic resonance imaging (MRI) scan at the level of the cerebellum demonstrating a filling defect (arrow) within the right transverse sinus consistent with cerebral venous thrombus.

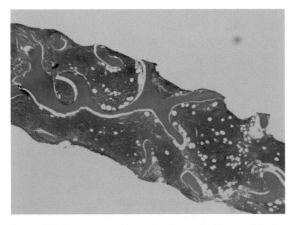

Figure 133 Bone marrow biopsy showing marked hypercellularity and an increased number of megakaryocytes.

KEY POINT

In the absence of the kinase mutation a bone marrow aspirate and biopsy will help to make the diagnosis of ET. Hypercellularity and an increase in megakaryocyte numbers are often present. Megakaryocyte morphology (appearances) is often abnormal and an increase in marrow fibrosis may be present.

What is the differential diagnosis of the headache?

There are many causes. In a woman of this age migraine, muscle spasm, fibromyalgia, temperomandibular malocclusion and sinusitis would be common. In older patients, temporal arteritis, cervical disc degeneration, spondylosis and cluster headaches need to be considered.

Venous sinus thrombosis and subarachnoid, subdural and epidural bleeding may all produce headache. Brain tumours, primary and secondary, are always a consideration.

In view of the headache and the elevated platelet count, what further investigations should be undertaken?

A magnetic resonance imaging (MRI) scan of the brain. A hypercoagulable screen to rule out any congenital coagulation defect that could predispose her to thrombosis. The most common congenital defect is factor V Leiden which slightly increases the risk of thrombosis; however, in the absence of other factors such as cigarette smoking and the oral contraceptive pill, it is unlikely to cause cerebral thrombosis. An antinuclear antibody screen, lupus anticoagulant and anticardiolipin antibody testing should be carried out. Patients with lupus erythematosus can present for the first time with thrombotic events (cerebral or others).

Contrast-enhanced MRI at the level of the cerebellum demonstrates a filling defect within the right transverse sinus consistent with cerebral venous thrombosis (Fig. 134).

The tests for lupus and hypercoagulable states were negative.

> **KEY POINT**
>
> Although patients with ET are prone to thrombotic episodes it is not clear that this thrombotic event caused the patient's symptom of headache. Headache is a common symptom in patients with ET although it is rarely caused by an intracranial vascular event.

What is the likely diagnosis?

The most likely diagnosis is ET in view of the elevated platelet count, abnormal platelet morphology, bone marrow appearances and lack of any other diagnosis. The absence of the *JAK2* mutation does not negate the diagnosis, as it is only found in 50% of cases.

What is the approach to treatment?

The treatment of ET is controversial. In young patients with a platelet count of $<1000 \times 10^9/L$ many clinicians would treat with aspirin 75 mg/day alone provided there are no complicating factors such as hypertension, smoking, oral contraceptive use or other congenital or acquired hypercoagulable disorders or a previous thrombotic event.

In patients with platelet counts of $>1000 \times 10^9/L$ treatment should be commenced to reduce the platelet count. There are no specific platelet-lowering agents available at present so a choice is made between hydroxyurea, an antimetabolite, and anagrelide, a phosphodiesterase inhibitor, which inhibits maturation from megakaryocytes into platelets.

Both agents have drawbacks. Hydroxyurea is a form of chemotherapy and is teratogenic. It reduces the haemoglobin and white cell count. One study suggests it might cause acute leukaemia after prolonged use.

Anagrelide is well tolerated in young patients but a recent study suggests it may increase the rate of bone marrow fibrosis. It causes vasodilatation and therefore a reflex tachycardia may occur causing unpleasant palpitations.

Interferon is effective but its chronic use is made difficult because of toxicity and the requirement for a daily subcutaneous injection.

Maria was treated with low molecular weight heparin and hydroxyurea and both were well tolerated. A Mirena coil was inserted as a contraceptive. Her headache disappeared. Maria's platelet count returned to $194 \times 10^9/L$.

Maria was discharged to her family doctor on warfarin and hydroxyurea but returned 3 months later saying she wished to become pregnant.

How should Maria be managed?

Hydroxyurea should be stopped before pregnancy. Folic acid supplementation should be given to reduce the risk of neural tube defects. Warfarin should be stopped when pregnancy is confirmed and low molecular weight heparin substituted.

Can you now construct an algorithm for the diagnosis of a high platelet count?

Yes.

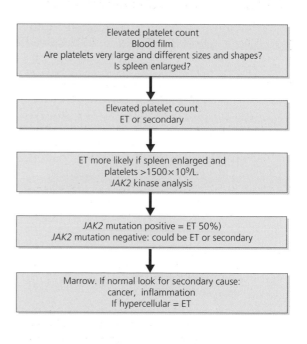

Outcome. Medication was changed as outlined above and Maria had a successful pregnancy and delivered a healthy boy weighing 4 kg.

CASE REVIEW

With current access to blood counts for family doctors it is now common for patients with high platelet counts to be identified before symptoms are present. In this case the abnormal finding was detected by the blood transfusion service. This is a very useful function of the blood transfusion service and asymptomatic conditions are occasionally identified which can be diagnosed and treated at an early stage of the disease.

The finding of a high platelet count is usually pathological unless the individual has had a splenectomy. The challenge for the doctor is to decide whether this represents a primary Myeloproliferative disorders (MPD) or a secondary phenomenon. The physical examination may reveal an enlarged spleen which shifts the probability to an MPD. Frequently, as in this case, there are no specific physical signs.

A very important investigation is a careful examination of the blood film by an experienced observer. The presence of large and abnormal looking platelets usually heightens the suspicion of an MPD such as ET. Secondary causes of thrombocytosis (an elevated platelet count) usually result in an increased number of platelets in the blood film but the appearance of the platelets is often normal. The major concern in older patients is an occult cancer. The search should include a careful physical examination to include breast and prostate as primary sources and a rectal examination with determination of the presence of occult bleeding. A chest radiograph in a smoker is mandatory. In the event of negative symptoms and signs of cancer sophisticated investigations are probably not warranted.

This young woman had ET and the real challenge is to prescribe the correct treatment. Currently, there are no specific agents that are aimed at reducing the platelet count specifically. The choice of therapy will depend on the age of the patient and concurrent pathological conditions, e.g. hypertension, a prior thrombotic event, a coincidental hypercoagulable state.

KEY POINTS

- MPDs are relatively uncommon in young people and their incidence rises as the age of the population increases.
- Until recently there was no specific test to identify patients with ET from those with a secondary cause of thrombocytosis. The suspicion for many years was of an intracellular defect that made the blood cells, in this case the megakaryocytes, hypersensitive to the usual growth factors in the bone marrow. A number of investigators have recently described an acquired genetic defect, a mutation, which results in uninhibited cell proliferation (Case 16). Although the identification of the kinase mutation is virtually diagnostic of ET, in the appropriate clinical setting, the test is positive in only about 50% of cases

- A clinical history, physical examination and appropriate investigations are still required in most patients undergoing investigation for a high platelet count. In the absence of the molecular kinase mutation there is no specific diagnostic test of ET
- Thrombocytosis can be secondary to chronic inflammation (e.g. chronic inflammatory bowel disease), bleeding or hyposplenism and is seen in MPD and ET
- A number of clinical trials are currently underway to identify drugs that will specifically be aimed at the kinase mutation (e.g. imatinib, an abl tyrosine kinase inhibitor in CML; Case 10) and hopefully they will prove to be effective, specific and non-toxic

Further reading

Baxter EJ, Scott LM, Campbell PJ, *et al.* Acquired mutations of the tyrosine kinase JAK2 in human myeloproliferative disorders. *Lancet* 2005; **365**: 1054–1061.

Kralovics R, Passamonti F, Buser AS, *et al.* A gain-of-function mutation of JAK2 in myeloproliferative disorders. *New England Journal of Medicine* 2005; **352**: 1779–1790.

Skoda R. The genetic basis of myeloproliferative disorders. asheducationbook.hematologylibrary.org/cgi/content/full/2007/1/1 Accessed in 2007.

Tefferi A & Gilliland G. Classification of myeloproliferative disorders: from Dameshek towards a semi-molecular system. *Best Practice and Research. Clinical Haematology* 2006; **19**: 365–385.

Tefferi A, Thiele J, Orazi A, *et al.* Proposals and rationale for revision of the World Health Organization diagnostic criteria for polycythemia vera, essential thrombocythemia and primary myelofibrosis: recommendations from an ad hoc international expert panel. *Blood* 2007; **110**: 1092–1097.

PART 2: CASES

Case 22   A 68-year-old man with a headache and confusion

Jose de Almagro, a 68-year-old retired journalist, was brought to the accident and emergency department of the local hospital. He lived alone and was unaccompanied. Jose's neighbour had noticed that he was confused when she brought him his daily newspaper. He was not sure what day it was and said he had a severe headache. He was unable to give a clear history but says that his urine has been red for a few days and his headache was getting worse. Jose was unable to give his full address and thought he was taking a number of medications but could not remember their names and had not brought them with him.

What should be done?

Ask Jose for his wallet or any other document he might have that contains his name and address. Try to find out if he has a relative or somebody who can provide a more complete history.

Carry out a full physical examination including a neurological examination.

Jose has ecchymoses on his arms and backs of his hands and an irregular pulse. The rate was 95 per minute and it was 'irregularly irregular'. His blood pressure was elevated at 180/120 mmHg.

He continues to complain of severe headache during the examination. His cranial nerves are intact and there are no localizing signs. His fundi showed mild arterio-venous (AV) nipping but no haemorrhages.

What is your differential diagnosis?

The pulse is the main clue. Jose probably has atrial fibrillation because he has an irregularly irregular pulse rate with a mild tachycardia. He could have multiple atrial

Haematology: Clinical Cases Uncovered. By S. McCann, R. Foà, O. Smith and E. Conneally. Published 2009 by Blackwell Publishing, ISBN: 978-1-4051-8322-2

ectopic beats, atrial tachycardia or a junctional tachycardia.

The headache suggests meningitis, viral or bacterial, or an intracranial or subarachnoid haemorrhage.

What should be done next?

Take an electrocardiogram (ECG) tracing and examine his urine for the presence of blood in view of his history and physical findings.

Jose's ECG tracing shows atrial fibrillation (Fig. 135) and mild left ventricular hypertrophy. There is no evidence of recent infarction. There are no P waves, numerous F waves and irregular ventricular contractions.

The dipstick indicated the presence of blood in his urine.

KEY POINT

The dipstick detects the presence of haemoglobin in the urine but does not differentiate between red blood cells and free haemoglobin. A microscopic examination will detect the presence of red cells.

How can you connect the atrial fibrillation, ecchymoses, haematuria and a possible subarachnoid or intracranial haemorrhage?

Jose has atrial fibrillation although the cause is not clear. He is probably taking warfarin to prevent emboli and may have exceeded the dose or taken some medication that has potentiated the action of warfarin.

What should be done next?

In view of the possibility of warfarin ingestion a coagulation screen including an international normalized ratio (INR) should be undertaken as an emergency.

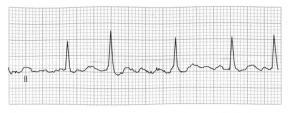

Figure 135 Electrocardiogram (ECG) showing atrial fibrillation. Absent P waves and irregular ventricular depolarization.

Table 62 Results of the coagulation tests.

	Patient's results	Normal range
PT	>99 s	12.0–15.0 s
APPT	>130 s	26.0–35.0 s
INR	>8.7 s	Only patients taking warfarin

APPT, activated partial thromboplastin time; INR, international normalized ratio; PT, prothrombin time.

What tests are routinely carried out in a coagulation screen and why would you request an INR?

The prothrombin time (PT) and the activated partial thromboplastin time (APPT). The platelet count does not affect either of these tests. The INR was developed and standardized for patients on vitamin K antagonists such as warfarin. The INR standardizes PT measurement based upon the characteristics of the thromboplastin reagent used by the laboratory and thus allows direct comparisons of INRs generated by different thromboplastins used in different laboratories in any given patient taking warfarin. See Table 62.

Now what is your differential diagnosis?

The grossly prolonged PT and APPT suggest a deficiency of a number of coagulation factors. This could certainly be explained by ingestion of the most likely drug, warfarin.

Other diagnoses in an adult would be an acquired inhibitor, disseminated intravascular coagulation (DIC), but this would usually be to a single coagulation factor such as factor VIII which would not prolong the PT. Rarely, B-cell neoplasms such as multiple myeloma or Waldenström's macroglobulinaemia can produce an

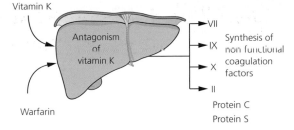

Figure 136 Mechanism and site of action of warfarin.

immunoglobulin that inhibits multiple coagulation factors. Pan-acting inhibitors with lupus anticoagulant for example can affect FVIII, IX, XI and XII but normally don't cause bleeding.

The coagulation tests and clinical findings are compatible with a diagnosis of anticoagulant overdose.

> **KEY POINT**
>
> The National Patient Safety Agency, UK (NPSA-UK) has recommends that patients carry a warfarin alert card in their wallet.

What is warfarin and how does it work?

Warfarin is structurally related to vitamin K. It is bound to albumin in the plasma. Warfarin inhibits the carboxylation of clotting factors II, VII IX and X and thus inhibits their binding to activated membranes and acting as clotting factors. However, the synthesis of these inactive factors continues and they are known as PIVKAs (proteins induced by vitamin K absence). The mechanism and site of action is shown in Fig. 136.

How long does it take, after ingestion, for warfarin to exert its anticoagulant action?

The half-lives of factors II, VII, IX and X are different and the inactivation by warfarin will therefore be time dependent (Fig. 137).

> **KEY POINT**
>
> The majority of patients taking warfarin are elderly and confusion about the dose taken, or taking other medications that potentate warfarin, are common causes of bleeding.

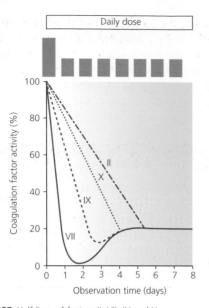

Figure 137 Half-lives of factors II, VII, IX and X.

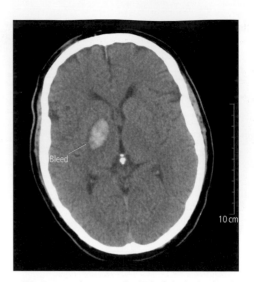

Figure 138 Computed tomography (CT) of the brain showing an intracerebral haemorrhage.

Warfarin is metabolized in the liver by cytochrome P450 2C9 system which also metabolizes many other drugs, making drug interactions a problem.

The common drugs that potentiate the anticoagulant effect of warfarin are azole antibiotics, macrolides, quinolones, non-steroidal anti-inflammatory drugs, including selective cyclo-oxygenase-2 inhibitors, selective serotonin reuptake inhibitors, omeprazole, lipid lowering agents and amiodarone.

> **KEY POINT**
>
> Co-administration of these drugs with warfarin should be avoided or closely monitored.

What factors influence the incidence of anticoagulant overdose?

The intensity of anticoagulation, concomitant clinical disorders and age. Patients <65 years without risk factors have a 3% chance of having a significant bleed, whereas this figure rises to 42% in patients over 65 with multiple risk factors.

What are the known risk factors that increase the risk of bleeding while taking warfarin?

A past history of stroke, gastrointestinal bleeding, myocardial infarction, anaemia, renal failure or diabetes mellitus. Elderly patients may also have an increased sensitivity to warfarin and should receive reduced doses compared to younger patients. Other disorders such as dementia may result in the patient taking the wrong dose of the drug inadvertently.

What should be done next?

Order an emergency CT/MRI of the brain and ask for a neurosurgical consultation.

The axial CT shows high attenuation in the right basal ganglia consistent with an acute intracerebral haemorrhage (Fig. 138).

While waiting for the radiological investigation and the neurological consultation what steps should be taken to correct the coagulation abnormality and stop the bleeding?

Vitamin K (10 mg IV) should also be given immediately. Infusions of plasma products such as fresh frozen plasma (FFP) and/or prothrombin complex concentrates (PCC). PCC provides the most rapid replacement of vitamin K-dependent factors and is the treatment of choice providing a superior clinical outcome compared to FFP for patients with intracranial bleeds. However, it should be remembered that although infusions of plasma products usually result in a rapid reversal of anticoagulation

Table 63 The ideal international normalized ratio (INR) will depend on the reason for the anticoagulation.

Indication	Target INR
Pulmonary embolus	2.5
Proximal deep vein thrombosis	2.5
Calf vein thrombosis	2.5
Recurrence of VTE: off warfarin	2.5
Recurrence of VTE: on warfarin	3.5
Symptomatic inherited thrombophilia	2.5
APLS	2.5
Non-rheumatic atrial fibrillation	2.5
Atrial fibrillation caused by rheumatic heart disease, congential heart disease, thyrotoxicosis	25
Cardioversion	2.5 or 3.0
Mural thrombus	2.5
Cardiomyopathy	2.5
Mechanical valve: aortic	2.5 or 3.0
Mechanical valve: mitral	3.5 or 3.0
Bioprosthetic valve	2.5 if anticoagulated

APLS, antiphospholipid syndrome; VTE, venous thromboembolism.

within minutes, it takes up to 1 hour to have these products ready for administration as they have to be thawed beforehand. Their effect is transient as the half-life of FVII is only 4–6 hours (Table 63) and therefore repeated infusions will be necessary especially if neurosurgical intervention is warranted.

Recent recommendation from the British Committee for Standards in Haematology (BCSH) is that for a major bleed 5–10 mg vitamin K IV and PCC are given.

What did the neurosurgeon advise?
She advised that Jose should be stabilized and when the INR had returned to normal she would review him again.

What recently discovered factors have been shown to influence the patient's response to warfarin?
A number of well-described genetic polymorphisms (dif-

ferences) have been discovered that influence the rate of metabolism of warfarin. There are three main alleles of CYP2C9 and patients may be homozygous or heterozygous. The maintenance dose of warfarin required will vary depending on the CYP2C9 allele present and the daily dose may vary from 1.5 mg to over 5 mg.

> **KEY POINT**
>
> Many patients who in the past were thought to comply poorly with the dosage of warfarin prescribed are now known to have a CYP2C9 polymorphism.
>
> VKOR1C mutations may also cause warfarin resistance and different alleles have been shown to affect the induction dose of warfarin. There is a wide variation in the prevalence of different alleles in different racial groups.

For what length of time should a patient be anticoagulated?
This depends on the reason for the anticoagulation. Some conditions require life-long anticoagulation. Patients with venous thromboembolism (VTE) require anticoagulation for 3–6 months. Prolonged administration reduces the risk of recurrence of VTE, but increases the risk of bleeding. Those with bioprosthetic heart valves, should receive warfarin for 3 months and those with mitral valve disease, a mechanical valve or atrial fibrillation require warfarin for life.

When deciding to anticoagulate a patient the doctor commonly begins with heparin, which has an immediate action. How should you change a patient from heparin to warfarin?
Begin warfarin concomitantly with heparin. Give heparin for 5 days as it takes this amount of time (96 hours) for warfarin to exert its maximum anticoagulant effect (even though the INR is prolonged before this). When INR is in the desired range for two consecutive days stop the heparin.

If you wish to start a patient on warfarin without giving heparin is there any advantage to giving a loading dose?
Not really. Begin with 5 mg (2 mg in the elderly or frail).

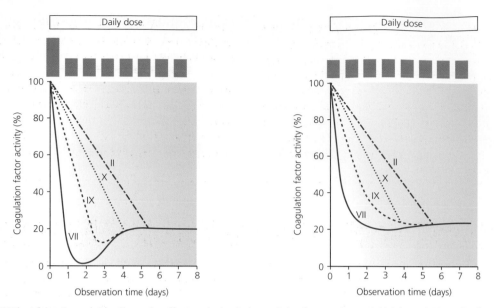

Figure 139 Chart for anticoagulation. Shows the effect on the level of coagulation factors when an initial dose of 10 mg (loading dose) or 5 mg is given.

Educate the patient and titrate the dose of warfarin until the INR is in desired range. Monitor INR daily initially and then weekly. If rapid anticoagulation is necessary begin with 10 mg on day one (Fig. 139).

Outcome. In spite of correcting the INR the intracranial bleed extended and Jose died the next day.

Can you now construct an algorithm for a patient who presents with spontaneous bleeding?

Yes.

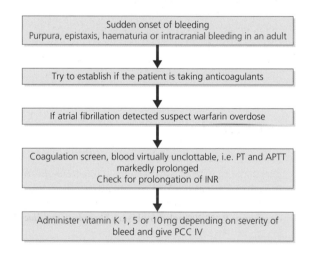

CASE REVIEW

An elderly patient is brought into the A&E who is confused and bleeding. This is a common problem. The difficulty in making a diagnosis is compounded by a lack of history and the absence of a friend or relative to give an accurate account of the problem. This is a problem of increasing frequency in our modern urbanized society.

Faced with this emergency the physical examination proves vital and the presence of atrial fibrillation immediately alerts the doctor to the possibility of warfarin

Continued

overdose, as patients with a known history of atrial fibrillation will be treated with warfarin indefinitely.

An assessment of the extent of the bleeding plus rapid action to correct the coagulation abnormality is of equal importance. The correction of the coagulation abnormality in this situation is difficult and the doctor must restore normal haemostasis as rapidly as possible without making the patient 'hypercoagulable' which could lead to embolic phenomena. There is no possibility of surgery until the coagulopathy is corrected.

In spite of monitoring, the problem of bleeding is significant especially in elderly patients. Remember 20% of serious bleeding episodes are fatal in this population. A number of things may make the doctor wary of prescribing warfarin, such as a history of bleeding, protein C or S deficiency, vitamin K deficiency, alcohol abuse and dementia.

As in this case there is commonly no helpful history and in spite of rapid corrective action fatal bleeds still occur.

KEY POINTS

- The variability in INR results in patients taking warfarin may be because of genetic polymorphisms and have nothing to do with patient compliance. Unfortunately, at present we have no easy method of diagnosing CYP2C9 or VKOR1C polymorphisms to guide us with anticoagulant dosing.
- Certain patients may require life-long administration of warfarin apart from those mentioned above. Patients with inherited thrombophilia (e.g. antithrombin deficiency), antiphospholipid syndrome, recurrent idiopathic VTEs, cancer, thrombotic pulmonary hypertension and certain patients may require anticoagulation during pregnancy.

Warfarin cannot be used during pregnancy as it crosses the placenta and is teratogenic. Although very widely used in all countries warfarin can cause skin necrosis, microembolism, agranulocytosis, diarrhoea, nausea and anorexia.

- Two new drugs, a direct thrombin inhibitor and an anti Xa have been licensed for the prevention of DVT and should receive a licence for atrial fibrillation. The advantages of these drugs will be a standard dose and no requirement for laboratory monitoring.

Further reading

Baglin TP, Keeling DM, Watson HG; British Committee for Standards in Haematology (BCSH). Guidelines for oral anti-coagulation (warfarin): 3rd edition – 2005 update. *British Journal of Haematology* 2005; **132**: 277–285.

Hoffe JV, Johnson FB, Longtine J, *et al*. Warfarin dosing and cytochrome P 450 209 polymorphisms. *Thrombosis and Haemostasis* 2004; **91**: 1123–1128.

Li T, Chang CY, Jin DY, *et al*. Identification of the gene for vitamin K epoxide reductase. *Nature* 2004; **427**: 541–544.

Tanube J, Halsall D & Boglin TG. Influences of cytochrome P-450 CYP2C9 polymorphisms on warfarin sensitivity and risk of overanticoagulation in patients on long-term treatment. *Blood* 2000; **96**: 1816–1819.

Case 23 · A 10-year-old boy with a fever

Milos Koniček, a 10-year-old boy said to his mother that he was feeling unwell following a game of football. She took his temperature and found it to be 38°C. She gave him antipyretic and analgesics and put him to bed. The next day she brought Milos to the family doctor, as he was still feeling unwell, tired and had a persistent fever.

Physical examination revealed pallor but no other abnormality.

What is your differential diagnosis?

A fever in a young boy has a very wide differential diagnostic possibility including infection, (viral and/or bacterial) or autoimmune disease. Localizing signs are usually apparent in the case of infection.

As there were no abnormal physical findings, apart from pallor, the doctor asked the mother and Milos to return if the fever had not resolved or if any new symptoms became obvious.

In 1 week she returned with Milos because the fever had persisted and he still felt unwell. Again pallor was the only physical sign.

What should be done?

Because of the persistent symptom and signs of pallor and fever the doctor should suspect something serious in a child of this age. The doctor should conduct a complete physical examination and order some simple blood tests.

The blood test results were available the following day. The blood count results are shown in Table 64. Some of the lymphocytes were described as having a 'blast-like' appearance.

Now what is your differential diagnosis?

Milos is anaemic and leucopenic, with a low neutrophil count. The lymphocyte count is at the lower limit of normal and some abnormal mononuclear cells are seen. The platelet count is reduced. Milos probably has a significant blood disease.

The differential diagnosis should include aplastic anaemia, Fanconi's anaemia, Gaucher's disease, Niemann–Pick disease, very severe infections, paroxysmal nocturnal haemoglobinuria and acute leukaemia.

What should be done next?

Because of the possibility of a serious blood disease Milos should be referred to a specialist immediately. The family doctor should advise that both parents accompany the child.

What should the specialist do?

Repeat the history and physical examination; carry out a biochemical screen and a bone marrow aspirate in view of the possibility of a serious blood disease.

The biochemical screen revealed an elevated lactic dehydrogenase (LDH) of 950 IU/L (normal range for a child 230–600 IU/L).

KEY POINT

LDH is a ubiquitous enzyme present in all cells and is released into the plasma when cells die. It is elevated in many haematological disorders including ineffective erythropoiesis, haemolysis and leukaemia.

Before carrying out the blood test and bone marrow what should the specialist tell the boy and his parents?

The specialist should reassure Milos that he will not feel any pain and he needs to examine the 'factory' where the

Haematology: Clinical Cases Uncovered. By S. McCann, R. Foà, O. Smith and E. Conneally. Published 2009 by Blackwell Publishing, ISBN: 978-1-4051-8322-2

Table 64 Results of the blood test.

	Patient's results	Normal range (female)
Hb	10.5 g/dL	11.5–16.4 g/dL
MCV	90.0 fL	83–99 fL (μm^3)
MCH	29.0 pg/cell	26.7–32.5 pg/cell
MCHC	32.0 g/dL	30.8–34.6 g/dL
WBC	2.0×10^9/L	$4.0–11.0 \times 10^9$/L (10^3/μL)
Platelets	100×10^9/L	$140–450 \times 10^9$/L (10^3/μL)
Neutrophils	1.0×10^9/L	$2.0–7.5 \times 10^9$/L (10^3/μL)
Lymphocytes	1.0×10^9/L	$1.5–3.5 \times 10^9$/L (10^3/μL)

Hb, haemoglobin; MCH, mean corpuscular haemoglobin; MCHC, mean corpuscular haemoglobin concentration; MCV, mean corpuscular volume; WBC, white blood cell count.

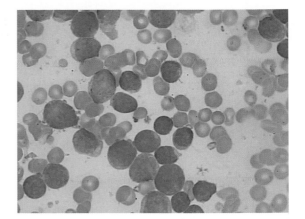

Figure 140 A bone marrow showing numerous 'blasts' without any normal myeloid or red cell precursors.

blood is made (the bone marrow). He should tell Milos' parents that he suspects acute leukaemia but that in the majority of cases, in children, this disease is now curable.

How is a bone marrow specimen obtained in a 10-year-old child?

Milos should be admitted to the hospital and the following blood tests should be requested: blood count, biochemical screen and coagulation screen.

Serum urate and lactic dehydrogenase are critical parameters in the event of a high white cell count. The sudden lysis of leukaemia cells may cause hyperuricaemia and impair renal function (tumour lysis syndrome).

An anaesthetist should review Milos and his family, and a specific consent for general anaesthesia should be requested. The doctor who will perform the procedure should obtain a separate consent.

Milos should be accompanied to the operating room together with one of his parents and a nurse. The parent remains in the operating room until Milos has been fully sedated. The anaesthetist will tell the doctor when he can proceed. The doctor uses an aseptic technique (sterile gloves, disinfection of skin, sterile needles preparation).

Using the first drops of marrow obtained with a small syringe (2 mL), slides are prepared to study the cellular

morphology by light microscopy. With a larger syringe (5 mL), approximately 4 mL of marrow should be drawn for further studies.

The marrow showed a reduction in the normal myeloid, erythroid and megakaryocytic elements (which explains pancytopenia) and an 80% replacement with leukaemia blasts (Fig. 140).

Now what is the likely diagnosis?

The marrow appearances are diagnostic of acute leukaemia. Other possibilities include neuroblastoma, rhabdomyosarcoma, Ewing's sarcoma and medulloblastoma.

What further tests should be carried out and why?

A number of further investigations are carried out in specialist laboratories in order to make a precise diagnosis of the type of leukaemia. These tests are designed to identify the 'lineage' and level of differentiation of the leukaemia cells. This identification also provides a prognostic guide to the doctor and the parents, and influences the specialist to pick the most appropriate therapy to effect a cure.

Cytochemistry and flow cytometry are the first tests to be performed and can be carried out in a very short time (minutes for cytochemistry, hours for flow cytometry). Cytochemistry showed that the leukaemic cells were myeloperoxidase (MPO) negative and periodic acid–Schiff (PAS) positive. This is strongly indicative of an acute lymphoblastic leukaemia (ALL).

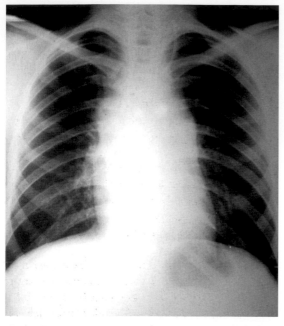

Figure 141 A chest radiograph showing a large mediastinal mass in a child with T-cell acute lymphoblastic leukaemia (ALL).

The flow cytometry characterization indicated that the blasts had an immunophenotypic profile diagnostic of a B-lineage ALL and, in particular, of a common ALL: TdT⁺ (early lymphoid marker), CD19⁺ (B-cell marker), CD10ᶦ (common ALL antigen), CD7⁻/CD3⁻ (T-cell markers), CD13⁻/CD33⁻ (myeloid markers).

For further details of flow cytometry see Part 1.

> **KEY POINT**
>
> Common acute lymphoblastic leukaemia – as indicated by the word – is the most frequent subtype of ALL, accounting for about 70–80% of cases both in children and in adults. In common ALL, blasts show a block in B-cell differentiation. A less common form is characterized by a block in T-cell differentiation and is commonly accompanied by a mediastinal (thymic) mass (Fig. 141).

Which other tests need to be carried out and why?

Cytogenetic and molecular analyses are carried out in order to identify if specific genetic markers are present. These may have important prognostic and therapeutic implications. A typical example is the Philadelphia (Ph) chromosome frequently found in adults with B-lineage ALL and less frequently recorded in child-hood disease. Ph+ ALL are enrolled in therapeutic programs that include tyrosine kinase inhibitors (Case 10).

What should the specialist tell the child and the parents?

The specialist should inform the parents that the suspicion of acute leukaemia has indeed been confirmed and that their child has common ALL. This is the most frequent type of leukaemia in childhood and is generally associated with a good outcome. This means that Milos should be admitted immediately to hospital to start treatment immediately. They should also know that further tests will be performed on the leukaemic cells in order to further define the characteristics of the blasts (see below).

The specialist will also have to inform Milos, together with his parents, that the marrow is not perfect and this is the reason for the fever and for the changes in his blood values. This will require hospitalization and treatment to put things right. It will have to be explained to Milos that to prevent more serious infections, he will have to stay in hospital for some time and that the number of persons he can see will have to be limited (see below).

> **KEY POINT**
>
> This is one of the most difficult points in the early management of children with acute leukaemia. Unlike adults, they are generally well and find themselves 'isolated' from one day to another, while the day before they were at school, playing football (as for Milos). The collaboration of the parents and staff is essential. News has to be given gradually. The word 'leukaemia' should not be used initially (Milos is 10); it will become clear over time. The meaning of chemotherapy and the issue of hair loss (a considerable problem for girls) should both be mentioned but not immediately after hospitalization. In many paediatric settings, psychological support is operational, multimedia facilities are available and school is organized in the ward, to give the impression that usual life has not been interrupted.

What type of acute leukaemia is most common in children compared with adults?

ALL is the most common form in children, while in adults acute myeloid leukaemias (AML) predominate.

Apart from the cell of origin of the leukaemias, what is the main difference between acute leukaemia in adults and children?

The majority of children with ALL are cured (approximately 80%), whereas in adults cure rates are about 40% and vary widely with age.

Is leukaemia a common disease in children?

No. Leukaemia is a relatively rare disease, occurring in about 2 in 100,000 of the population. However, ALL represents the most frequent cancer in childhood.

KEY POINT

As in adults, acute leukaemia most probably is an acquired genetic disease. In the majority of cases it is sporadic, but occasionally it occurs in more than one member of a family. Studies in identical twins, in archived neonatal blood spots of patients and in normal newborn cord bloods suggest that chromosomal translocations often initiate leukaemia prenatally (before birth). The disease appears to represent a malignancy of bone marrow stem cells.

What specific abnormalities influence the outcome?

The total white cell count (WBC) still influences the outcome and the probability of long-term cure. The higher the WBC the worse the outlook. The low WBC frequently observed in children with ALL is one of the reasons for the more favourable outcome compared to adults, in whom the counts are usually increased (greater tumour burden).

Leukaemia involving the meninges (lining of the brain) is not uncommon so a lumbar puncture with careful examination of the cerebrospinal fluid (CSF) in a specialist laboratory is essential. If leukaemia cells are found in the CSF then intensive intrathecal chemotherapy is given.

How is a lumbar puncture carried out in children?

Intrathecal chemotherapy (methotrexate injected into the spinal fluid) is usually given to prevent brain relapse while the child is asleep.

What is the approach to treatment?

In the majority of cases a combination of corticosteroids and chemotherapy is recommended. Once the disease is no longer detectable, a programme of maintenance chemotherapy is undertaken. All children receive some form of prophylaxis (preventive medication) to prevent future development of meningeal involvement.

What is the likely impact on the child and his parents?

Unfortunately, the treatment of the leukaemia will cause Milos to be quite ill initially. Treatment causes damage to the normal bone marrow cells resulting in a further fall in haemoglobin, neutrophils and platelets before marrow recovery occurs and the leukaemia is eradicated. There may be a requirement for red cell and platelet transfusions, and large doses of antibiotics. Milos may require the placement of a semi-permanent device implanted under the skin to make recurrent transfusions less traumatic. He will miss school and contact with friends and may become depressed. Physical appearance may change as a result of therapy. Significant parental stress is common and this may impose great strain on a marriage. Because of the need for repeated intravenous chemotherapy and transfusions a number of options are available to make venous access easier for Milos (Fig. 142).

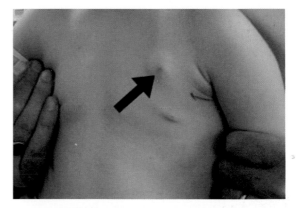

Figure 142 A Portacath device implanted under the skin (arrow) in a child with acute lymphoblastic leukaemia (ALL) to facilitate intravenous access.

PART 2: CASES

KEY POINT

Treatment to eradicate ALL always includes large doses of corticosteroids. This produces toxicity, which can be disfiguring and occasionally life-threatening. Common toxicities include weight gain, hyperglycaemia, hypokalaemia, hypertension, peptic ulceration, striae in the skin of the abdomen and, less frequently, psychotic episodes. Avascular necrosis of the head of the femur may also occur.

Can you now construct an algorithm for the diagnosis of fever, pallor and fatigue in a child?

Yes.

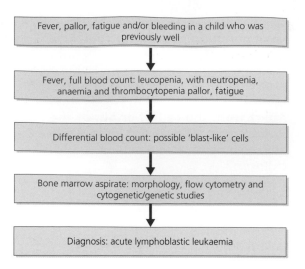

Fever, pallor, fatigue and/or bleeding in a child who was previously well

↓

Fever, full blood count: leucopenia, with neutropenia, anaemia and thrombocytopenia pallor, fatigue

↓

Differential blood count: possible 'blast-like' cells

↓

Bone marrow aspirate: morphology, flow cytometry and cytogenetic/genetic studies

↓

Diagnosis: acute lymphoblastic leukaemia

CASE REVIEW

In most cases, children who present with a fever, sore throat or feeling generally unwell have a benign disease, usually a viral or bacterial infection. Therefore it is difficult for the primary care physician to suspect leukaemia or a related disorder, as these are relatively rare diseases.

With easy and rapid access to blood counts the diagnostic problem has become less difficult although many children will not like providing a blood sample. The findings of neutropenia and anaemia in this case were a clue that there was a serious underlying disorder to explain the boy's symptoms and signs. The majority of children with ALL present with a neutropenia and in many cases there are no abnormal cells in the blood film. The differentiation between abnormal cells and lymphocyte variants (seen in viral infection) requires an experienced observer.

Neutropenia should always be taken seriously and investigated (for variation in blood counts in different races see Part 1a).

Rapid referral to a specialist is essential as the correct diagnosis, accompanied by expert treatment, usually results in cure. Unfortunately, the child and his/her parents often experience huge stress, schooling is missed and interaction with peers may be a problem.

Although the majority of children are cured, it appears that some of them may experience minor problems such as difficulty with abstract thought such as mathematics in adulthood.

In children with disease that fails to respond to chemotherapy (a small minority) allogeneic stem cell transplantation may be curative.

KEY POINTS

- Although the diagnosis of ALL fills the patient and his/her parents with fear, the majority of children are cured. There is a heavy social price to pay for both the patient and his/her parents
- Accurate diagnosis and expert treatment by a specialist team influences the outcome
- New diagnostic techniques, such as 'gene profiling', may help to make the diagnosis more accurate and stimulate the development of new treatments with less toxicity
- A concept of minimal residual disease (MRD) has emerged. This means that we can use sophisticated laboratory techniques to detect 'minimal amounts' of leukaemia in the patient's blood or bone marrow when

they appear to be in 'complete remission'. The detection of this so-called MRD allows us to change our treatment strategy and to decrease or increase the 'strength' of the treatment
- Because of the success of treatment, attention is now focused on reducing treatment in appropriate patients in order to minimize toxicity without compromising cure rates
- A rare type of acute leukaemia in children is Burkitt's leukaemia/lymphoma. Burkitt made the original observation of a lymphoma in African children, and proposed that an infectious agent caused the disease. The lymphoma in Africa and the form of leukaemia worldwide carries his name and are caused by the Epstein–Barr virus.

Further reading

Arcesi R, Hann IM, Smith OP, eds. *Paediatric Haematology*, 3rd edn. Blackwell Publishing, 2006.

Earle EA & Eiser C. Children's behaviour following diagnosis of acute lymphoblastic leukaemia: a qualitative longitudinal study. *Clinical Child Psychology and Psychiatry* 2007; **12**: 281–293.

Greaves MF & Wiemels J. Origins of chromosome transloca-tions in childhood leukaemia. *National Reviews of Cancer* 2003; **9**: 639–649.

Hoffbrand AV, Moss PAH & Pettit JE. *Essential Haematology*, 5th edn. Blackwell Publishing, Oxford, 2006: 157–173.

Linker C, Sallan S, Gokbuget N & Pui C-H. Acute lymphoblastic leukemia in adults and children. asheducationbook.hema-tologylibrary.org 2006. Accessed in 2006.

For each situation choose the single option you feel is most correct.

> **1** *A young girl presents to the doctor with fatigue. She is otherwise asymptomatic. He finds that she is anaemic.*

Which of the following is the most likely cause of her anaemia?
a. Folate deficiency
b. Haemolysis
c. Iron deficiency
d. Vitamin B_{12} deficiency
e. Anaemia of chronic disease

> **2** *An elderly woman is brought to the clinic by her husband. He says her gait is unsteady and her memory is poor. She is mildly icteric and slightly agitated. She has pancytopenia.*

Which of the following is the most likely diagnosis?
a. A brain tumour
b. Acute leukaemia
c. Folate deficiency
d. Vitamin B_{12} deficiency
e. Aplastic anaemia

> **3** *A middle-aged man presents with shortness of breath and has signs of heart failure and jaundice. He is anaemic with a Hb of 5.0 g/dL and an MCV of 110 fL (μm^3). He has spherocytes on his blood film.*

Which of the following is the most likely diagnosis?
a. Iron deficiency anaemia

b. Autoimmune haemolytic anaemia
c. Vitamin B_{12} deficiency
d. Hereditary spherocytosis
e. Acute leukaemia

> **4** *A young boy of African descent presents with respiratory failure and has a Hb of 6.0 g/dL.*

Which of the following is the most likely diagnosis?
a. Hb C disease
b. Hb SA (sickle cell trait)
c. Hb SS (sickle cell disease)
d. β Thalassaemia major
e. α Thalassaemia

> **5** *A patient with hereditary spherocytosis presents to the clinic with a history of sudden onset of shortness of breath on exertion. He is noted to have pancytopenia.*

Which of the following is the most likely diagnosis?
a. An acute gastointestinal tract bleed
b. Acute leukaemia
c. Vitamin B_{12} deficiency
d. A drug allergy
e. An aplastic crisis secondary to parvovirus B19 infection

> **6** *A 67-year-old non-smoking patient presents because his wife said his colour was very 'high'.*

Which of the following is the most likely diagnosis?
a. Haemochromatosis
b. Thalassaemia
c. Vitamin B_{12} deficiency
d. Polycythemia vera
e. Chronic obstructive pulmonary disease (COPD)

Haematology: Clinical Cases Uncovered. By S. McCann, R. Foà, O. Smith and E. Conneally. Published 2009 by Blackwell Publishing, ISBN: 978-1-4051-8322-2

7 *A measurement of serum erythropoietin reveals an elevated result.*

Which of the following is the most likely diagnosis?
a. Polycythemia vera
b. Renal failure
c. Erythrocytosis secondary to hypoxaemia
d. Heart failure
e. An isolated renal cyst

8 *A 78-year-old man is found to have a lymphocytosis of 60×10^9/L.*

Which of the following is the most likely diagnosis?
a. Pertussis
b. Chronic myeloid leukaemia
c. Lung cancer
d. Chronic lymphoblastic leukaemia
e. Acute myeloid leukaemia

9 *A young boy has a fever and a white cell count of 35×10^9/L with anaemia and a low platelet count.*

Which of the following is the most likely diagnosis?
a. Aplastic anaemia
b. Chronic myeloid leukaemia
c. Acute lymphoblastic leukaemia
d. Acute myeloid leukaemia
e. Infectious mononucleosis

10 *Denis Burkitt is famous because of which of the following statements?*

a. He was the first person to describe leukaemia
b. He was the first person to devise a treatment for leukaemia
c. He was the first person to use chemotherapy
d. He was the first person to describe cancer caused by a virus
e. He was the first person to describe cancer caused by bacteria

11 *Which of the following statements is most likely to be true?*

a. Warfarin is only available intravenously
b. Warfarin is only available orally
c. Warfarin is excreted in the urine unmetabolized
d. Warfarin interferes with platelet function
e. Warfarin has very few drug–drug interactions

12 *A 72-year-old woman has a diagnosis of pernicious anaemia (vitamin B_{12} deficiency).*

Which of the following statements is most likely to be true?
a. The lactic dehydrogenase (LDH) is very high
b. The LDH is very low
c. The potassium rises after treatment
d. The reticulocyte count is elevated at diagnosis
e. The platelet count is high at diagnosis

13 *A 56-year-old man has anaemia and a positive Coombs' test (direct antiglobulin test).*

Which of the following statements is most likely to be true?
a. The reticulocyte count will be low
b. The reticulocyte count will be high
c. The erythrocytes will appear normal on the blood film
d. Iron stores will be decreased
e. The bilirubin will be normal

14 *A 68-year-old man has back pain and renal failure.*

Which of the following is the most likely diagnosis?
a. Lung cancer
b. Glomerulonephritis
c. Osteoporosis
d. Osteomalacia
e. Multiple myeloma

15 A 70-year-old woman has a diagnosis of multiple myeloma.

Which of the following statements is most likely to be true?
a. Immunoglobulins will be normal
b. A polyclonal gammopathy will be present
c. A monoclonal gammopathy will be present
d. The Hb will be normal
e. The ESR will be normal

16 A 46-year-old man presents with sudden onset of shortness of breath and haemoptysis.

Which of the following is the most likely diagnosis?
a. A pulmonary embolus
b. Lung cancer
c. A myocardial infarct
d. A pneumothorax
e. An intrapulmonary haemorrhage

17 A 25-year-old woman has anaemia. Her MCV, MCH and MCHC are all low.

What is the most likely diagnosis?
a. Vitamin B_{12} deficiency
b. Folic acid deficiency
c. The anaemia of chronic disease
d. Sickle cell disease
e. Iron deficiency

18 A 50-year-old man is diagnosed as having chronic myeloid leukaemia.

Which of the following karyotypic abnormalities is most likely?
a. An abnormal chromosome 3
b. A large chromosome 22
c. A reciprocal translocation between chromosome 7 and 22
d. A reciprocal translocation between chromosomes 9 and 22
e. Trisomy 21

19 Which of the following statements is most likely to be true?

a. Abnormal chromosomes are commonly found in acute leukaemias
b. Abnormal chromosomes are never found in acute leukaemias
c. Trisomy 3 is the most common abnormality found in acute leukaemias
d. Chromosome analysis is of no help in making a diagnosis of the type of leukaemia
e. Chromosome analysis is of no help in picking the most appropriate form of therapy for acute leukaemia

20 In a patient with iron deficiency anaemia which of the following statements is likely to be true?

a. The serum iron is the best test to confirm the diagnosis
b. The total iron binding capacity (TIBC) is the best test to confirm the diagnosis
c. An examination of the bone marrow is mandatory
d. A serum ferritin of <10 µg/L (ng/mL) is diagnostic of iron deficiency
e. Pica is common in adults

21 A 21-year-old woman is told she has coeliac disease.

Which of the following statements is most likely to be true?
a. She must have had a history of childhood diarrhoea
b. She will be of short stature
c. She may have iron deficiency anaemia
d. She will have vitamin B_{12} deficiency
e. She could not have folic acid deficiency

22 A 57-year-old woman has a platelet count of 1050×10^9/L and blood film shows platelet anisocytosis (different shapes).

Which of the following is the most likely diagnosis?
a. A gastrointestinal tract bleed
b. Lung cancer
c. Iron deficiency
d. Essential thrombocythaemia
e. Hypersplenism

23 *Which of the following products are not made from human blood?*

a. Recombinant factor VIII concentrates
b. Packed red cells
c. Cryoprecipitate
d. Granulocyte transfusions
e. Platelet concentrates

24 *Severe haemolytic transfusion reactions still occur in spite of precautions by the transfusion service.*

Which of the following statements is most likely to be true?
a. The most like cause is a laboratory error in blood grouping
b. The most likely cause is undetected HLA antibodies
c. Only occur in women who have had pregnancies
d. Never occur in women who have had pregnancies
e. Are caused by human error in giving the wrong blood which has not been cross-matched for the patient

25 *A 23-year-old woman has a large mediastinal mass and a diagnosis of Hodgkin's disease is made.*

Which of the following statements is most likely to be correct?
a. Her condition is likely to be curable
b. Her condition is likely to be incurable
c. She requires an allogeneic stem cell transplant
d. This is a highly contagious disease
e. She requires immediate splenectomy

26 *A 71-year-old man has multiple myeloma.*

Which of the following statements is most likely to be true?
a. His serum calcium will be normal
b. His serum calcium will be raised
c. His alkaline phosphatase will be raised
d. He will have osteoclastic lesions in his bones

27 *A 12-year-old boy has haemophilia A (low factor VIII).*

Which of the following statements is most likely to be true?
a. His father has haemophilia
b. His sister must be a carrier of the defective gene
c. His sister can never be a carrier of the defective gene
d. His mother is a carrier of the defective gene
e. His brother must have haemophilia

28 *A 35-year-old woman has acute myeloid leukaemia.*

Which of the following statements is most likely to be true?
a. Her full blood count is normal
b. Her platelet count is low
c. She has marked lymphadenopathy and splenomegaly
d. She has a large mediastinal mass
e. She has a VIIth nerve paralysis

29 *A 28-year-old woman with autoimmune haemolytic anaemia (AIHA) has a sudden worsening of her anaemia and a fall in her reticulocyte count.*

Which of the following statements is most likely to be true?
a. She has become iron deficient
b. She has become vitamin B_{12} deficient
c. Her haemolysis is getting worse
d. Her haemolysis is getting better
e. She has developed folate deficiency

30 *A 27-year-old man has acute myeloid leukaemia and a high fever.*

Which of the following statements is most likely to be true?
a. His fever is caused by his leukaemia
b. He should have blood cultures taken and the result awaited
c. He should have blood cultures taken and given broad-spectrum antibiotics immediately
d. He should be given aspirin to reduce his fever
e. If he has an infection the site will be obvious

EMQs

1 Causes of anaemia

a. Iron deficiency anaemia

b. Anaemia of chronic disease

c. Thalassaemia

d. *Helicobacter pylori* disease

e. Vitamin B_{12} deficiency

f. Folate deficiency

g. Hereditary spherocytosis syndrome

h. Autoimmune haemolytic anaemia

i. Aplastic anaemia

j. Acute leukaemia

k. Multiple myeloma

For each of the patients described below choose the most likely explanation for the anaemia from the above list. Each cause may be chosen once, more than once or not at all.

1. A 22-year-old woman with a history of recurrent jaundice is noted to have anaemia and a palpable spleen.

2. A 65-year-old man presents with fatigue, jaundice and splenomegaly. He is in mild heart failure.

3. A 35-year-old man with a history of coeliac disease presents with anaemia.

4. A 65-year-old woman who has had a gastrectomy (removal of her stomach) 30 years ago presents with anaemia.

5. A 75-year-old man complains of severe back pain, which is worse at night. He has had two episodes of anaemia in the last year. He is anaemic.

2 Examination

a. Splenomegaly

b. Jaundice

c. Pallor

d. Koilonychia

e. Lymphadenopathy

f. Petechiae

g. Haemarthrosis

h. Heart failure

i. Dorsal kyphosis

j. Rheumatoid arthritis

k. An enlarged liver

For each of the patients whose examination findings are described below choose the most likely diagnosis from the list above. Each diagnosis can be chosen once, more than once or not at all.

1. A 40-year-old woman with iron deficiency anaemia.

2. A 65-year-old man with a history of chronic lymphocytic leukaemia and autoimmune haemolytic anaemia.

3. A man with fatigue and arthritis. He has gynaecomastia and is very 'tanned'.

4. A young boy with a history of severe aplastic anaemia.

5. A 60-year-old woman with autoimmune haemolytic anaemia.

3 History

a. Pernicious anaemia

b. Coeliac disease

c. Thalassaemia

d. Autoimmune haemolytic anaemia

e. Iron deficiency anaemia

f. Polycythaemia (erythrocytosis)

g. Recurrent pneumonia

h. Chronic myeloid leukaemia

i. Heart failure

j. Recurrent jaundice

k. A family history of 'too much iron'

Haematology: Clinical Cases Uncovered. By S. McCann, R. Foà, O. Smith and E. Conneally. Published 2009 by Blackwell Publishing, ISBN: 978-1-4051-8322-2

For each of the patients whose history is described below choose the most likely diagnosis from the list above. Each diagnosis may be chosen once, more than once or not at all.

1. A 68-year-old man who has been a heavy cigarette and cigar smoker all his adult life. His wife says his colour is very 'high' recently.
2. A man who has chronic leukaemia and has a karyotype (chromosome analysis) showing a translocation between chromosomes 2 and 21.
3. A 30-year-old woman with a diagnosis of hereditary spherocytosis.
4. A 55-year-old man with recent onset of diabetes mellitus and arthritis.
5. A woman who has anaemia in all her five pregnancies.

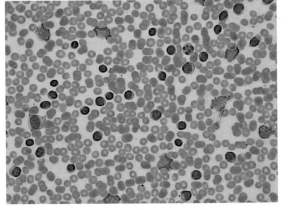

Film 2

4 Interpretation of blood film

a. Iron deficiency
b. Hereditary spherocytosis
c. Acute leukaemia
d. Autoimmune haemolytic anaemia
e. Vitamin B_{12} deficiency
f. Chronic lymphocytic leukaemia
g. Multiple myeloma
h. Thalassaemia
i. Sickle cell disease
j. Anaemia of chronic disease
k. Chronic myeloid leukaemia

For each patient whose blood film is shown below choose the most likely diagnosis from the list above. Each diagnosis may be chosen once, more than once or not at all.

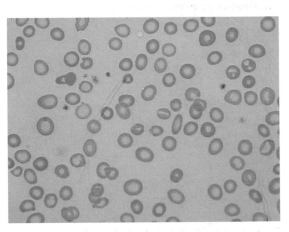

Film 3

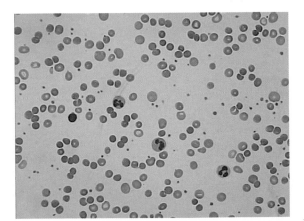

Film 1

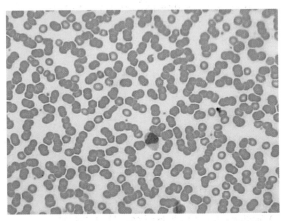

Film 4

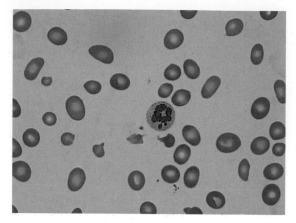

Film 5

5 Blood transfusion

a. Iron overload
b. Alloantibodies to red cell antigens
c. Autoantibodies to red cell antigens
d. Hepatitis C infection
e. HLA antibodies
f. A history of receiving a previous blood transfusion
g. A history of previous pregnancies
h. West Nile virus
i. Malaria
j. Pneumococcal pneumonia

For each of the patients whose history is described below choose the most likely diagnosis from the list above. Each diagnosis may be chosen once, more than once or not at all.

1. A 25-year-old woman from Sardinia with thalassaemia.
2. A 50-year-old woman with multiple red cell alloantibodies.
3. A 61-year-old man with haemolytic anaemia and a positive direct antiglobulin test (Coombs').
4. A 64-old woman with abnormal liver blood tests who received a red cell transfusion in 1987.
5. A man with a fever after receiving a red cell transfusion.

6 Interpretation of investigations

a. Autoimmune haemolytic anaemia
b. Pernicious anaemia
c. Iron deficiency anaemia
d. Chronic lymphocytic leukaemia
e. Sickle cell disease
f. Folate deficiency
g. Hereditary spherocytosis syndrome
h. Thalassaemia
i. Multiple myeloma
j. Haemochromatosis
k. Chronic myeloid leukaemia

For each of the patients whose investigations are described below choose the most likely diagnosis from the list above. Each diagnosis may be chosen once, more than once or not at all.

1. A 27-year-old woman with the following blood indices: Hb 9.0 g/dL, MCV 65 fL (μm^3), MCH 19 pg/cell, platelets 600×10^9/L.
2. An 80-year-old man with the following blood indices: Hb 13.5 g/dL, platelets 400×10^9/L, WBC 85.00×10^9/L with 90% lymphocytes.
3. A 70-year-old man with back pain and the following blood indices: Hb 10.00 g/dL, MCV and MCH normal, platelets 100×10^9/L. Blood film showed marked rouleaux formation.
4. A 5-year-old girl with the following blood indices: Hb 5.0 g/dL, MCV 62 fL (μm^3), WBC and platelets normal. Reticulocytes 500×10^9/L (upper limit 100×10^9/L).
5. A 62-year-old woman with the following blood indices: Hb 8.00 g/dL, normal WBC and platelets. Reticulocytes 250×10^9/L. Direct antiglobulin test (Coombs') test positive.

7 Clinical evaluation and interpretation of investigations

a. Haemoptysis
b. Haematemesis
c. Haematuria
d. Melaena
e. Haemarthrosis
f. Purpura
g. Petechiae in skin
h. Icterus
i. Anaemia
j. Cyanosis
k. Bone pain

For each of the patients whose investigations are described below, choose the most likely diagnosis from the list above. Each diagnosis may be chosen once, more than once or not at all.

1. A 60-year-old man who is taking warfarin for atrial fibrillation.
2. A 55-year old man taking aspirin.
3. A 20-year-old woman with a platelet count of 10×10^9/L.
4. A 70-year-old man with a diagnosis of lung cancer.
5. A 45-year-old man with coeliac disease.

---

8 Clinical evaluation and interpretation of investigations

a. Lymphocytosis in a 70-year-old man
b. Granulocytosis and splenomegaly in a 50-year-old man
c. Generalized lymphadenopathy and splenomegaly in a 70-year-old man
d. Splenomegaly and anaemia in a 5-year-old girl from Sardinia
e. Massive splenomegaly and anaemia in a 68-year-old man
f. Lymphadenopathy and a monocytosis in a 17-year-old girl
g. Lymphadenopathy, a mediastinal mass and lymphopenia in a 20-year-old woman
h. Splenomegaly, anaemia and icterus in a 58-year-old woman

For each of the patients whose investigations are described below, choose the most likely diagnosis from the list above. Each diagnosis may be chosen once, more than once or not at all.

1. Thalassaemia
2. Chronic myeloid leukaemia
3. Myelofibrosis
4. Hodgkin's disease
5. Infectious mononucleosis

---

9 Clinical evaluation and interpretation of investigations

a. Hepatosplenomegaly and a bronze skin in a 50-year-old man
b. A ferritin level of >1000 µg/L (ng/mL) in a 50-year-old man
c. A ferritin of 10 µg/L (ng/mL) in a 50-year-old man

---

d. A 70-year-old man with bone pain and a dorsal kyphosis
e. A 70-year old man with renal failure and a monoclonal gammopathy
f. A 70-year-old man with bone pain and recurrent chest infections
g. A 70-year-old man with melaena
h. A 70-year-old man with pancytopenia
i. A 70-year-old man with fever, weight loss and generalized lymphadenopathy

For each of the patients whose investigations are described below, choose the most likely diagnosis from the list above. Each diagnosis may be chosen once, more than once or not at all.

1. Haemochromatosis
2. Iron deficiency
3. Multiple myeloma
4. Acute myeloid leukaemia
5. Non-Hodgkin's lymphoma

---

10 Interpretation of investigations

a. A prolonged prothrombin time (PT)
b. A prolonged activated partial thromboplastin time (APTT)
c. A platelet count of 10×10^9/L
d. A platelet count of 1000×10^9/L
e. A factor VIII level of <1%
f. A prolonged APTT and a normal PT
g. A prolonged PT and a normal APTT
h. Recurrent haemarthroses in a 3-year-old boy
i. Haemarthroses in a 3-year-old girl
j. A shortened PT
k. Hb of 20 g/dL

For each of the patients whose investigations are described below, choose the most likely diagnosis from the list above. Each diagnosis may be chosen once, more than once or not at all.

1. Immune thrombocytopenic purpura (ITP)
2. Haemophilia
3. Polycythaemia vera
4. Essential thrombocythaemia
5. Lung cancer

SAQs

1 *A 75-year-old woman comes to the accident and emergency department complaining of fatigue and she noticed that she had been jaundiced for the past week. She is pale and icteric. She has splenomegaly and her Hb is 5.0 g/dL.*

a. How severe is her anaemia? Explain your assessment. *(2 marks)*

b. Outline your immediate management of this patient. *(3 marks)*

c. Which three investigations would be most useful in this patient? Explain why. *(3 marks)*

d. How would you manage this patient after discharge to minimize the risk of her condition relapsing? *(2 marks)*

2 *A 40-year-old-man is referred to a haematologist complaining of fatigue. His Hb is 10.4 g/dL, MCV 65 fL and MCH 20.0 pg/cell.*

a. What type of anaemia does he have? *(1 mark)*

b. What is the differential diagnosis of this type of anaemia? *(2 marks)*

c. What investigations would you carry out? *(4 marks)*

d. What bacterial infection could explain his anaemia? *(1 mark)*

3 *A 37-year-old woman is brought to the accident and emergency department following a severe road traffic accident. She has multiple injuries and is bleeding. She is pale, sweating and has a tachycardia.*

a. Outline your immediate management of this patient. *(2 marks)*

b. A decision is made to give her a blood transfusion prior to surgery for her multiple injuries. What do you need to know about her? *(2 marks)* What blood tests are required? *(2 marks)*

c. What infections can be transmitted via a red cell transfusion? *(4 marks)*

d. What is the most likely cause of a fever during or after the transfusion? *(1 mark)*

4 *A patient with a known diagnosis of multiple myeloma is referred to hospital because he is dehydrated, confused and in pain.*

a. Outline your immediate management of this patient. *(2 marks)*

b. What is the most likely metabolic abnormality present? *(1 mark)*

c. What secondary biochemical abnormalities are likely? *(2 marks)*

d. How should his pain be managed? *(2 marks)*

Haematology: Clinical Cases Uncovered. By S. McCann, R. Foà, O. Smith and E. Conneally. Published 2009 by Blackwell Publishing, ISBN: 978-1-4051-8322-2

5 *A 79-year-old woman is admitted via the accident and emergency department. She is confused, icteric, in heart failure and clinically very anaemic. Investigations reveal a Hb of 3.1 g/dL, RBC 1.2 × 10¹²/L, MCV 120 fL, a bilirubin of 34 µmol/L (2.2 mg/dL).*

a. Outline your immediate management of this patient. *(1 mark)*
b. What is the most likely diagnosis from her clinical signs and preliminary blood findings? *(2 marks)*
c. What other biochemical finding is likely? *(1 mark)*
d. What problems can be anticipated from blood transfusion in this patient? *(2 marks)*

6 *A 7-year-old boy presented to the doctor with a limp and a fever. He was febrile without any localizing signs. The doctor suspected acute leukaemia and sent him to a haematologist who carried out a bone marrow examination.*

a. What type of acute leukaemia is most common in children? *(2 marks)*
b. What are the principles of treatment? *(2 marks)*
c. What should the parents be told about the probable outcome? *(2 marks)*
d. What type of leukaemia/lymphoma is caused by a virus? *(1 mark)*

7 *A 27-year-old woman presents with a sudden onset of bruising. There are no abnormal physical findings apart from the purpura. A full blood count reveals a platelet count of <10 × 10⁹/L with a normal white cell count and Hb.*

a. What is the differential diagnosis? *(1 mark)*
b. What is your immediate management of this patient? *(3 marks)*
c. The bone marrow aspirate shows normal numbers of megakaryocytes (platelet precursors) and no abnormal cells. How does this help to make a diagnosis? *(1 mark)*
d. What toxicity is associated with treatment? *(4 marks)* *(maximum number of marks is 4)*

8 *A 75-year-old man presents with fatigue, night sweats and generalized lymphadenopathy. He also has an enlarged spleen. He has a history of recurrent pneumonia. His blood count shows the following: Hb 13.0 g/dL, WBC 45.5 × 10⁹/L (90% lymphocytes) with a normal platelet count. A presumed diagnosis of chronic lymphocytic leukaemia (CLL) is made.*

a. What types of lymphocytes are found in the blood of patient's with CLL? *(1 mark)*
b. Why would he have recurrent infections? *(2 mark)*
c. If he suddenly developed anaemia and jaundice what would be the most likely explanation? *(2 marks)* What investigations would you carry out? *(2 marks)*
d. Is this disease curable? *(2 marks)*

9 *A 46-year-old man presents to the hospital with a history of night sweats, fever and a feeling of fullness in his left side. A blood count shows: Hb 14.0 g/dL, WBC 65.8 × 10⁹/L with myelocytes, metamyelocytes and nucleated red cells present. His platelet count is elevated at 600 × 10⁹/L.*

a. What is the most likely diagnosis? *(1 mark)*
b. What investigation would you perform and why? *(2 marks)*
c. Is any cause known for this disease? *(1 mark)*
d. What is the current approach to treatment and how has it altered in the last 10 years? *(2 marks)*

10 *A 60-year-old man was admitted to hospital with a sudden onset of chest pain, haemoptysis and dyspnoea. A diagnosis of pulmonary embolus was suspected.*

a. What investigations would you carry out? *(2 marks)*
b. If the investigation were positive how would you treat this patient? *(2 marks)*
c. What treatment would you give at discharge and afterwards? *(1 mark)*
d. How would you monitor the treatment and what influences the response to treatment? *(4 marks)*

MCQs answers

1. c	11. b	21. c
2. d	12. a	22. d
3. b	13. b	23. a
4. c	14. e	24. e
5. e	15. c	25. a
6. d	16. a	26. b
7. c	17. e	27. d
8. d	18. d	28. b
9. c	19. a	29. e
10. d	20. d	30. c

Haematology: Clinical Cases Uncovered. By S. McCann, R. Foà,
O. Smith and E. Conneally. Published 2009 by Blackwell
Publishing, ISBN: 978-1-4051-8322-2

1
1. g
2. h
3. a and f
4. a and e
5. k

2
1. c and d
2. a, b, e and k
3. k
4. c and f
5. a, b and h

3
1. f
2. 0, none of the above
3. j
4. k
5. b and e

4
1. d
2. f
3. a
4. g
5. e

5
1. a
2. b, f and g
3. c
4. d
5. h and i

6
1. c
2. d
3. i
4. h
5. a

7
1. a, b, c, d, f, i
2. b, d, i
3. c, f, g, i

4. i, k
5. i

8
1. d
2. b
3. e
4. g
5. f

9
1. a, b
2. c, g
3. d, e, f, h
4. h
5. h, i

10
1. c
2. b, e, f, h
3. k
4. d
5. a, b, d, j

Haematology: Clinical Cases Uncovered. By S. McCann, R. Foà,
O. Smith and E. Conneally. Published 2009 by Blackwell
Publishing, ISBN: 978-1-4051-8322-2

SAQs answers

1

a. She has severe anaemia because a Hb of <7.0 g/dL is called severe *(1 mark)*. She has a palpable spleen therefore she probably has an underlying haematological condition *(1 mark)*. *(1 mark for each correct answer, maximum 2 marks)*

b. First, establish whether she needs basic life support or not (ABC) *(1 mark)*. As she does not, the next step is to give general support with high flow oxygen *(1 mark)*. Establish an intravenous line *(1 mark)*, obtain a chest radiograph *(1 mark)* and an ECG *(1 mark)*. Arrange her admission to hospital *(1 mark)*.

c. Get a full blood count, blood film *(1 mark)*, reticulocyte count *(1 mark)* and Coombs' test *(1 mark)*. A blood count will provide the red cell, white cell and platelet counts and the blood film will provide information on any red cell abnormalities *(1 mark)*. A raised reticulocyte count will indicate haemolysis or bleeding *(1 mark)*. A Coombs' test will let you know if there are antibodies (IgG and/or complement) on the red cells, confirming a diagnosis of autoimmune haemolytic anaemia *(1 mark)*.

d. She should be maintained on corticosteroids *(1 mark)* and given folic acid indefinitely *(1 mark)*.

2

a. He has a microcytic hypochromic anaemia *(1 mark)*.

b. The differential diagnosis includes iron deficiency *(1 mark)*, the anaemia of chronic disease *(1 mark)* and thalassaemia *(1 mark)*. His ethnic group will help with the possible diagnosis as haemoglobin disorders are not found in Caucasians.

Haematology: Clinical Cases Uncovered. By S. McCann, R. Foà, O. Smith and E. Conneally. Published 2009 by Blackwell Publishing, ISBN: 978-1-4051-8322-2

c. Faecal occult blood *(1 mark)*, OGD *(1 mark)*, colonoscopy *(1 mark)*, tTG antibody titre *(1 mark)*. This test is s sensitive marker of coeliac disease.

d. *Helicobacter pylori* can cause inflammation or ulceration leading to blood loss but can also cause iron deficiency by as yet unknown mechanisms *(1 mark)*.

3

a. Establish airway, assess breathing and circulation *(1 mark)*. Site an intravenous line *(1 mark)*.

b. You need to establish her identity and have a wrist band, bar coded, put on *(1 mark)*. You need to enquire about prior pregnancies (not births) or blood transfusions *(1 mark)*. Blood tests include a full blood count, LRB and group and cross-match *(2 marks)*.

c. Bacterial (rarely), viral, parasitic and prion *(4 marks)*.

d. A non-haemolytic transfusion reaction caused by contaminating white blood cells (WBC) (if blood has not been leukodepleted) of cytokine release from WBC *(1 mark)*.

4

a. Assess his hydration status (skin turgor, eyeball pressure) *(1 mark)* and immediately establish an intravenous line and begin a normal saline infusion *(1 mark)*.

b. In a patient with multiple myeloma the most likely abnormality is hypercalcaemia. This leads to confusion, polyuria and severe dehydration *(1 mark)*.

c. Hypercalcaemia causes calcium deposition in the kidney and together with the dehydration and possible deposition of immunoglobulin light chains gives rise to a raised creatinine *(2 marks)*.

d. Opiate analgesia should be given parenterally. It is important to mobilize patients with multiple myeloma as quickly as possible. Adequate pain relief is a prerequisite for mobilization *(2 marks)*.

5

a. Give her oxygen and establish intravenous access *(1 mark)*.

b. Vitamin B$_{12}$ deficiency caused by pernicious anaemia. These patients can have a very low Hb which is tolerated because of the insidious onset. The red cell count is low because of ineffective erythropoiesis and the MCV is elevated *(2 marks)*.

c. Because of the ineffective erythropoiesis the lactic dehydrogenase (LDH) is grossly elevated (sometimes so high it is unrecordable) *(1 mark)*.

d. Because of her age, heart failure and probable low blood volume it is possible to precipitate more severe heart failure and even death by rapid blood transfusion. These patients are best treated by vitamin B$_{12}$ replacement *(2 marks)*.

6

a. In children the predominant type of leukaemia is lymphoblastic (ALL) *(2 marks)*. Although uncommon, acute myeloid may also occur and the outcome is not as good.

b. The principles of treatment are repeated courses of combination chemotherapy including high doses of corticosteroids until complete remission is obtained and then 'maintenance therapy', mostly as an outpatient, for 2 years *(1 mark)*. Because of the risk of leukaemia in the meninges, prophylaxis is given with intrathecal drugs *(1 mark)*.

c. In most cases of childhood ALL the child is cured *(1 mark)*. There may be mild impairment of some cerebral function, such as mathematical skills, in later life *(1 mark)*.

d. The Epstein–Barr virus causes Burkitt's leukaemia/ lymphoma. The endemic form of this disease was first described by Burkitt in equatorial Africa and Papua New Guinea. Unfortunately, the search for viruses as a cause of the common varieties of acute and chronic leukaemias has been unsuccessful thus far.

7

a. In the absence of any physical findings (especially an enlarged spleen) and any symptoms a diagnosis of immune thrombocytopenia *(1 mark)* is likely in this age group and gender. Other causes of thrombocytopenia include drugs, leukaemia, bone marrow infiltration, bone marrow failure syndromes (e.g. aplastic anaemia) and other autoimmune diseases such as systemic lupus erythematosus (SLE).

b. Admit her to hospital. Check for retinal haemorrhages *(1 mark)*. Make sure she is not given aspirin or non-steroidal anti-inflammatory drugs *(1 mark)* and that all medications are given by mouth or intravenously *(1 mark)*.

c. Normal numbers of megakaryocytes, in the absence of any other abnormality in the bone marrow, together with a low platelet count makes the diagnosis of immune thrombocytopenia very likely as in this condition platelet lifespan is markedly reduced *(1 mark)*.

d. Treatment of immune thrombocytopenia consists of high dose corticosteroids initially. Toxicities include hyperglycaemia *(1 mark)*, hypokalaemia *(1 mark)*, hypertension *(1 mark)*, psychosis *(1 mark)*, *Candida* infection in the mouth, oesophagus and vagina *(1 mark)*.

8

a. In normal individuals T cells predominate in the blood. Chronic lymphocytic leukaemia (CLL) is a disease of B cells *(1 mark)*.

b. Patients with CLL commonly have hypogammaglobulinaemia *(1 mark)* and therefore are subject to recurrent infections. A combination of reduced antibody responses and reduced opsonization *(1 mark)* contribute to this.

c. A sudden drop in Hb in the absence of bleeding is commonly caused by autoimmune haemolysis *(1 mark)*. The jaundice is caused by the hyperbilirubinaemia secondary to the haemolysis *(1 mark)*. A reticulocyte count should be performed to assess the marrow's capability of responding to the haemolysis *(1 mark)* and a Coombs' test should be carried out to confirm the diagnosis of autoimmune haemolysis. The Coombs' test detects antibody and/or complement bound to the red cell membrane *(1 mark)*.

d. Combination chemotherapy, when indicated, can bring the disease into remission but relapse is inevitable in most patients *(1 mark)*. A small number of young patients may be cured with stem cell transplantation *(1 mark)*.

9

a. This blood picture and the symptoms and signs make the diagnosis of chronic myeloid leukaemia (CML) almost a certainty *(1 mark)*.

b. A cytogenetic analysis, karyotype *(1 mark)* or fluorescence *in situ* hybridization (FISH) analysis

(1 mark), looking for the Philadelphia chromosome (small chromosome 22) (karyotype) or the reciprocal translocation between chromosomes 9 and 22, t(9:22) (FISH). This acquired genetic abnormality is present in all patients with CML *(1 mark)*.

c. The only cause we know is exposure to high doses of ionizing radiation *(1 mark)*. The dropping of the atomic bombs on Japan during the Second World War resulted in many deaths from CML.

d. The current approach is to use tyrosine kinase inhibitors *(1 mark)* and a response is expected in most patients. This has replaced allogeneic stem cell transplantation as front line therapy for most patients *(1 mark)*.

10

a. Pulse oxymetry *(1 mark)* and a CT pulmonary angiogram *(1 mark)*. This has replaced ventilation–perfusion scans as it is easier to perform and more accurate *(1 mark)*.

b. If the pulmonary embolus was life-threatening and the diagnosis was made shortly after the onset of symptoms, thrombolysis should be undertaken *(1 mark)*. If not, the patient should be treated with low molecular weight or unfractionated heparin and warfarin *(1 mark)*.

c. He should be discharged on warfarin as the anticoagulant of choice *(1 mark)*.

d. He should be monitored with the international normalized ratio (INR) test *(1 mark)*. The level should be kept between 2.5 and 3.0 *(1 mark)*. There are a number of polymorphisms that influence the metabolism of warfarin *(1 mark)* and may lead to difficulties in optimizing the dose as there is no easy clinical test available at present *(1 mark)*.

Appendix: normal laboratory values and CD table

These values may vary from laboratory to laboratory and country to country, depending on the type of equipment used to carry out the assay and the population being tested. It is extremely important to check the reference values in the laboratory that is carrying out the test for your patient. The values given here have been obtained from the laboratory of St James' Hospital Dublin and are in common use in Europe. Results given in brackets are those commonly used in North America.

	Normal range (female)	Normal range (male)
Haemoglobin	11.5–16.4 g/dL	13.5–18.0 g/dL
Red blood cell count (RBC)	$4.0–5.2 \times 10^{12}$/L (10^6/µL)	$4.6–5.7 \times 10^{12}$/L (10^6/µL)
MCV	83–99 fL (µm³)	
MCH	26.7–32.5 pg/cell	
MCHC	30.8–34.6 g/dL	
Platelet count	$145–450 \times 10^9$/L (10^3/µL)	
White blood cell count (WBC)	$4.0–11.0 \times 10^9$/L (10^3/µL)	
Neutrophils	$2.0–7.5 \times 10^9$/L (10^3/µL)	
Lymphocytes	$1.5–3.5 \times 10^9$/L (10^3/µL)	
Monocytes	$0.2–0.8 \times 10^9$/L (10^3/µL)	
Eosinophils	$0.04–0.40 \times 10^9$/L (10^3/µL)	
Reticulocytes	$20–100 \times 10^9$/L (0.2–1.5%)	
Erythrocyte sedimentation rate (ESR)	0–15 mm/hour	0–10 mm/hour
Haptoglobin	0.45–2.05 g/L (30–220 mg/dL)	
Vitamin B_{12}	150–1000 ng/L (µg/mL)	
Red cell folate	150–1000 ng/L (pg/mL) of packed red cells	
Serum ferritin	20–300 µg/L (ng/mL)	
Transferrin saturation	<38%	
Erythropoietin (EPO)	6.0–25.0 mIU/mL	
Pulse oximetry: O_2 saturation	>96%	
Red cell mass	20–30 mL/kg	

	Normal range (female)	Normal range (male)
Plasma volume	40–50 mL/kg	
Total blood volume	60–80 mL/kg	
D-dimers	<500 ng/mL	
Fibrinogen	1.5–4.0 g/L	
Prothrombin time (PT)	12.0–15.0 seconds	
Activated partial thromboplastin time (APTT)	26.0–35.0 seconds	
Bilirubin	0–17 µmol/L (0.3–1.1 mg/dL)	
Direct bilirubin	0–7.0 µmol/L (0–0.3 mg/dL)	
Lactic dehydrogenase (LDH)	230–450 IU/L	
Aspartame amino transferase (AST; also SGOT)	7–40 IU/L	
Alkaline phosphatase	40–120 IU/L	
Gamma glutamyl amino transferase (GGT)	10–55 IU/L	
Fasting blood glucose	<7.0 mmol/L (<125 mg/dL)	
Potassium	3.5–5.0 mmol/L	
Calcium	2.30–2.70 mmol/L (8.8–10.8 mg/dL)	
Serum creatinine	50–115 µmol/L (0.5–1.3 mg/dL)	
Uric acid	150–470 µmol/L (3–8 mg/dL)	
Albumin	35–50 g/L (3.5–5.0 g/dL)	
Total protein	60–80 g/L (6.0–8.0 g/dL)	
IgG	6.40–15.22 g/L (700–1450 mg/dL)	
IgA	0.48–3.44 g/L (70–370 mg/dL)	
IgM	0.29–1.86 g/L (30–210 mg/dL)	

Male ranges as for females unless otherwise indicated.

CD TABLE

Name

CD2 T lymphocytes. E-rosette receptor
CD3 T-cell receptor
CD4 T helper lymphocytes
CD5 T lymphocytes
CD7 T lymphocytes
CD8 T suppressor/cytotoxic lymphocytes
CD19 B lymphocytes
CD20 B lymphocytes
CD22 B lymphocytes
CD23 B lymphocytes
CD56 NK lymphocytes
CD57 NK lymphocytes
CD52 All lymphocyte populations

Glossary

aetiology   cause of disease

allele   alternative form of DNA occupying a specific chromosomal locus

Alzheimer's   a degenerative disease of the central nervous system leading to dementia and memory loss

anaemia   the occurrence of Hb below the lower limit for the age and gender of the individual

angina   chest pain induced by myocardial ischaemia

anorexia   loss of appetite

apoptosis   a form of programmed cell death. It involves a series of biochemical events leading to a characteristic cell morphology and death

aspirate   removing of tissue through suction of a needle

ataxic   an uncoordinated gait (walk)

autologous stem cell graft   the use of stem cells from the individual to reconstitute haemopoiesis following myeloablative chemotherapy

autosomal recessive   a form of inheritance, which requires both alleles for manifestation of the effect

barrier method   condom/diaphragm

BFU-E   burst-forming unit erythroid. The term given to a colony of mature red cells growing after 14 days incubation from a human stem cell in the presence of erythropoietin

blind loop syndrome   overgrowth of bacteria in a stagnant loop of bowel

Caucasian   an individual of European extraction

CFU-E   colony-forming unit erythroid. The term given to a colony of mature red cells growing after 7 days' incubation from a human stem cell in the presence of erythropoietin

CFU-GEMM   a colony of erythroid cells, granulocytes and macrophages. The term given to a mixed colony growing from a human stem cell

CFU-GM   colony-forming unit, granulocyte, macrophage. The term given to a colony of granulocytes and macrophages growing from a human stem cell

CFU-MEG   colony-forming unit, megakaryocyte. The term given to a colony of mature megakaryocytes growing from a human stem cell

chelation   removal of iron from body tissues

chemotherapy   compounds that cause destruction (apoptosis) of malignant cells or infectious agents

chronic bronchitis   productive cough for more than 3 months recurring

cirrhosis   fibrotic chronic liver damage with regeneration

coagulopathy   deficiency of coagulation proteins leading to bleeding

coeliac	a disease caused by allergy to gluten resulting in villus atrophy and folate acid/iron malabsorption
complement	a complex series of proteins, which participate in the immune response
Crohn's disease	inflammatory disease usually of the distal small bowel
CSF	cerebrospinal fluid
cyst	a fluid-filled sac
cytokine	low molecular weight protein, which regulates the immune system, haemopoiesis and the inflammatory response
cytoskeleton	protein structure, which maintains cell shape
diverticulum	an outpouching of the mucosa and submucosa usually of the large bowel
embolus	thrombus (clot), which has moved along a blood vessel
emphysema	destruction of alveoli within the lung
erythropoiesis	synthesis of red cells
extensor plantar Babinski sign	an up-going big toe with fanning of the other toes following stroking of the lateral surface of the foot. Indicates an upper motor neurone lesion
extramedullary	outside the bone marrow
ferritin	a complex of iron and apoferritin. Small amounts are present in plasma and reflect body iron stores
fibrinogen	a soluble protein in plasma which is converted to fibrin (insoluble) by thrombin
gluten	a component of wheat
gout	an acute arthritis caused by deposition of uric acid crystals in the joints
granulocyte	neutrophil with granules in the cytoplasm
haemoglobin molecule	made up of four globin chains containing iron and responsible for oxygen transport
haemolysate	contents of destroyed red cells

haemopoietic	relating to the synthesis of the elements of the blood
haemopoietic stress	increased demand on the bone marrow to produce more cells
hepatic siderosis	deposition of iron in the liver
hepatosplenomegaly	enlargement of the liver and spleen
hypoxaemic	reduced oxygen saturation
immunoglobulin	glycoprotein synthesized by B cells (antibodies)
ineffective erythropoiesis	premature destruction of red cells within the bone marrow
intrathecal	into the CSF
intrauterine growth retardation	failure of fetus to develop normally
Jack Russell terrier	a small dog
karyotype (cytogenetics)	analysis of chromosomes
kyphosis	curvature of the spine secondary to collapse of a vertebral body
lymphadenopathy	enlargement of lymph nodes
lymphoma	malignant transformation of lymphocytes within lymph nodes
lymphoproliferative disease	malignant proliferation of lymphocytes in the blood/ marrow/lymph nodes
malaise	a feeling of fatigue
malaria	a disease caused by a parasite, which invades red cells and can cause severe haemolysis
matrix	semi-solid medium, which supports cellular growth
MCH	mean corpuscular haemoglobin (see Appendix)
MCHC	mean corpuscular haemoglobin concentration (see Appendix)
MCV	mean corpuscular volume (see Appendix)
mediastinum	above and anterior to the heart
megaloblastic	asynchronous development of nucleus and cytoplasm in the bone marrow caused by a deficiency of vitamin B_{12} or folic acid
menarche	occurrence of the first menstrual period

metabolism	build-up or breakdown of complex molecules
metastasis	spread of neoplastic cells to a distal site
midwife	nurse who takes care of women during pregnancy
moiety	a portion of a molecule
monoclonal	immunoglobulin/light chain derived from a single lymphocyte/plasma cell
monocyte	white cell with single nucleus and blue–grey cytoplasm, the circulation equivalent of tissue macrophages
myelin	a lipoprotein sheath that surrounds axons in the CNS
nausea	a feeling of sickness/desire to vomit
necrosis	a form of traumatic cell death that results from acute cellular injury
neonatologist	physician who looks after newborns
neoplasm	malignant proliferation
occult	not visible (hidden)
optic fundi	posterior part of the eye where small blood vessels are visible
osteoporosis	demineralization of bone
paraneoplastic	a syndrome occurring in association with malignancy but not a direct result of it
petechiae	pinpoint bleeding into the skin
phagocytic	engulfment and destruction of foreign material by white cells
pharyngeal web	a membrane occurring in the post-cricoid area of the pharynx in severe iron deficiency leading to development of malignant change
phlebotomy	removal of red cells from the circulation
plethoric	fullness caused by increased haemoglobin or blood flow
pneumothorax	collapse of lung because of air in the pleural space
polychromasia	blue–grey colour of young red cells
portal hypertension	increased blood pressure in the portal circulation usually caused by chronic liver disease
pre-eclampsia	a syndrome in pregnancy characterized by hypertension, proteinuria and oedema
prophylaxis	prevention
radionucleotide	a nucleotide labelled with radioactive material
radiotherapy	treatment of malignant disease by gamma rays or X-rays
remission	inability to detect disease following treatment
reticulocyte	young red cell which is able to synthesize small amounts of haemoglobin for 24–48 hours
reticuloendothelial	a widespread system within the body controlling in part immune response to infection
Rhesus	a blood group
ribosome	cellular structure in which protein synthesis occurs
sclera	the white of the eye
sickling	polymerization of Hb S within red cells
spina bifida	congenital lesion with failure to close the spinal cord associated with folate deficiency *in utero*
spontaneous abortion	loss of fetus not caused by external manipulation
tender	sore to touch
thrombophilia	inherited prothrombotic states
transcription factor (sometimes called a sequence-specific DNA binding factor)	a protein that binds to specific parts of DNA using DNA binding domains and is part of the system that controls the transfer (or transcription) of genetic information from DNA to RNA. Transcription factors perform this function alone, or by using other proteins in a complex, by increasing or preventing the presence of RNA polymerase, the enzyme that activates the transcription of genetic information from DNA to RNA

transferrin   a plasma protein that transports iron

tropical sprue   progressive mucosal injury to the small bowel probably caused by infection

unfixed   without the addition of formalin

units of alcohol   one unit is equivalent to ½ pint of beer or one measure of spirits

urinanalysis   microscopic and chemical examination of the urine

vascular dementia   dementia caused by reduced blood supply to the brain

venesection   removal of blood from a vein

Index of cases by diagnosis

Index